W0080246

# Educational Dimensions of School Lunch

Suzanne Rice • A. G. Rud
Editors

# Educational Dimensions of School Lunch

## Critical Perspectives

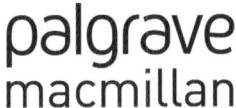

*Editors*
Suzanne Rice
University of Kansas
Lawrence, KS, USA

A. G. Rud
Washington State University
Pullman, WA, USA

ISBN 978-3-030-10218-0    ISBN 978-3-319-72517-8    (eBook)
https://doi.org/10.1007/978-3-319-72517-8

© The Editor(s) (if applicable) and The Author(s) 2018
Softcover re-print of the Hardcover 1st edition 2018
This work is subject to copyright. All rights are solely and exclusively licensed by the Publisher, whether the whole or part of the material is concerned, specifically the rights of translation, reprinting, reuse of illustrations, recitation, broadcasting, reproduction on microfilms or in any other physical way, and transmission or information storage and retrieval, electronic adaptation, computer software, or by similar or dissimilar methodology now known or hereafter developed.
The use of general descriptive names, registered names, trademarks, service marks, etc. in this publication does not imply, even in the absence of a specific statement, that such names are exempt from the relevant protective laws and regulations and therefore free for general use.
The publisher, the authors and the editors are safe to assume that the advice and information in this book are believed to be true and accurate at the date of publication. Neither the publisher nor the authors or the editors give a warranty, express or implied, with respect to the material contained herein or for any errors or omissions that may have been made. The publisher remains neutral with regard to jurisdictional claims in published maps and institutional affiliations.

Cover illustration: © Sam Stephenson / Alamy Stock Photo

Printed on acid-free paper

This Palgrave Macmillan imprint is published by Springer Nature
The registered company is Springer International Publishing AG
The registered company address is: Gewerbestrasse 11, 6330 Cham, Switzerland

*Dedicated to the memory of Matthew T. Lewis*

# FOREWORD

It stuns me sometimes to think about how central school feeding has become in worldwide politics and civic discussion, both in and out of the educational sphere. I have marveled to see widespread, often viral attention in the United States to issues like "pink slime," "pizza as a vegetable," and "lunch shaming." It seems nearly everyone is talking school lunch. A decade ago, when I began studying school food in earnest, there were a small but growing number of scholars—in educational research and in other fields like sociology (Poppendieck 2010) and history (Levine 2008)—and a growing number of teachers, administrators, school nutrition professionals, parents and concerned citizens who already took school food seriously. Yet that number has grown exponentially over the past two decades, spurred by exposés and documentaries like *Fast Food Nation* (Schlosser 2001), *The Omnivore's Dilemma* (Pollan 2006), *Food, Inc.* (Kenner 2008), and Jamie Oliver's television series on either side of the Atlantic (Gilbert and Walker 2005; Smith 2010), not to mention growing "crises" of obesity and diabetes, and high-profile politicians—US First Lady Michelle Obama perhaps most noticeably—pushing gardens and exercise and nutritional "nudges." All these tens of thousands of intellectuals, activists, public servants, and citizens have been taking seriously the policies and practices of the lunchroom; the implications for students, the environment, and animals; and the legacy we are creating for our culture and society. Not just in the United States, either, but transnationally, for school food makes headlines in the United Kingdom, Canada, Italy, Ghana, Australia, South Korea, Aotearoa New Zealand, and many more.

I first became acquainted specifically with the work of Suzanne Rice and A. G. Rud, editors of and contributors to this volume, in 2013, when reading a special issue of *The Journal of Thought* all about school lunch (Rice 2013). Just a couple of years before, I had published an essay titled "Why Educational Researchers Should Take School Food Seriously" (Weaver-Hightower 2011), and it was a delight to encounter these scholars who did in fact take school food seriously—as a critical part of education and society worthy of deep examination. Not only did they take it seriously, but they pushed on the boundaries of who the stakeholders of school food really are and, indeed, what the stakes are for getting school food right. It was immediately clear to me that the authors in that special issue would become important teachers for me about the politics and practices of school food.

That first introduction of mine to these important thinkers explains why I feel so honored to pen the foreword to their impressive collection you now hold, *Educational Dimensions of School Lunch: Critical Perspectives*. They and their contributors are scholars that continue to take seriously the need to research, rethink, and reform school food in multiple educational contexts. They have important new insights to share about the history, complexity, interconnectedness, and impact of a part of the school day that too many view as simple and inconsequential. This book arrives at a truly important time in our global history, when we face multiple and seemingly contradictory crises of hunger, unconscionable waste, and obesity. We face truly hard decisions about how to ethically, sustainably, and healthily feed the world. This book provides much-needed insights that push forward current discussions and policymaking.

This is a very philosophical volume. I don't mean that in any pejorative sense that it lacks practicality or grounding in the empirical life of schools. Quite the opposite. Rather, I see within these pages a deep, abiding interest in uncovering the ontology of why we feed children; the epistemology of classrooms, lunchrooms, off-campus fast food joints, lunchboxes, and homeschooler kitchens; and the ethics and morality of the choices about what (or who) we eat, where, when, and how reflectively we do so. Perhaps most especially one feels within the volume a yearning for aesthetics and love to return to school meals, for food to appeal to our senses rather than simply stuff our guts, for our foodways and eating spaces to inspire learning and connection rather than just impose obedience and efficiency.

Given that several of the contributors are well regarded in philosophy of education, one should not be surprised by this book's philosophical leaning. Still, it is a philosophical volume in that the authors stake claims and explore them, challenging readers to clarify—or perhaps regret—their own positions. We readers consider along the way our relationships to other animals, to gender, to growing things, to justice for our fellow citizens, to our abilities and disabilities, to racial histories and the racialized present, to the parental role of teachers, to the larger environment and its man-made destructions, to the curriculum we allow to be taught in our name, and to what is real versus merely spectacle. All of this intersects with food, of course, because food stands as perhaps the most basic part of human existence.

Importantly, the contributors also help us reconnect to past philosophers of education, restoring our collective memory that food has long been part of our most cherished thinkers' ideas about culture and learning. Rud and Gleason remind us of John Dewey's and Paulo Freire's notions of food as central to just and acculturative education. Laird notes Dewey's food-related philosophies, too, as well as those of Montessori, Steiner, and proponents of the kindergarten movement. Salvio uncovers the theoretical tensions for Margaret Mead, the great anthropologist of sexual practices and education in the South Pacific, as she later worked to set up the US government's first national nutrition policies. Remembering these histories can hopefully lead modern educators to restore food to the center of educational thinking in teacher education, educational leadership training, and the foundations of education.

*Educational Dimensions of School Lunch: Critical Perspectives,* as the subtitle implies, also delves deeply into the social justice of food. The authors escort us to the school gardens of Berkeley, California; to the food deserts of Detroit, Michigan; to a private school lunchroom in Kansas and one in a Midwestern city public school; into lunchboxes in Aotearoa New Zealand, Australia, and England; and to the school cafeterias that have become utterly surveilled "total institutions" (Goffman 1962). In these locales the authors take up the causes of the most vulnerable: the land, air, and water; animals; farm and slaughterhouse workers; the hungry and misnourished; those in food deserts; those from oppressed or marginalized cultures; those in developing nations; and, of course, the captive audience of students.

Naturally, the volume's contributors focus on the roles of school—the day-to-day phenomena of educating. That endlessly repeated process obviously installs the "what is" of food and foodways, which the contributors critique, ably showing readers *how* schools (wittingly or not) create technologies to keep students under control and unaware of how food is made. Crucially, though, the authors also imagine pedagogies and curricula of "what could be" within schools. Schools, each essay posits, are one way out of the mire of unhealthy, unjust, and unsustainable practices. This volume provides ample starting places for concerned professionals to become activists for better school food, better educational experiences for students, and a better society—for what Lupinacci and Happel-Parkins call "examples of curriculum and pedagogy that breathe life into the potential of diverse, socially-just, and sustainable communities." It is an educative stance, seeking *mindful* rather than *mindless* eaters.

The volume's contributors also do not fall into the lazy trap of simply suggesting schools add one more thing to the curriculum. Rather, they recognize well the ever-increasing pressure on educators to be everything to everyone, to roll with the intensification of curriculum standards and ever-expanding testing regimes, and to solve all of society's ills. Instead, these thoughtful scholars envision a food education that takes advantage of interdisciplinary curriculum, seizing moments—like lunch—often viewed as non-educative to engage students, and involving community partners in work related to schools and their communities.

Many things from these pages might stay with readers; I know they will for me. Stapleton and Cole's conversation, based in Cole's struggles to help hungry kids in her school, rivets the reader with its depictions of the daily operation of inequality in an urban alternative school. We leave that chapter convinced that food deserts are as real *inside* schools as they are outside them. Pluim, Powell, and Leahy's chapter recounts a similarly affecting story of Natia, a student who all around her are quick to hold up as the avatar of unhealthiness though they tragically overlook her poverty and hunger. It is a story hard to calm down after. I could point out similarly rich moments from every chapter.

Ultimately, as the authors you are about to encounter make clear, we fight so bitterly over school food because it is so multivalent, so layered with the deepest of meanings about what it is to be human, to take pleasure, to exercise self-restraint, to develop culture and identity, to be generous or stingy, to teach and learn, and to govern. *Educational Dimensions of School Lunch* maps this contested terrain wonderfully, casting light on some of the darkest, unseen corners of the school lunchroom. Better still, the contributors lead us not to paralysis, but instead they argue vehemently—and correctly, to my mind—that explicit teaching about food holds the power to transform not only what appears on children's noontime trays but also the very future of our planet and our societies.

Educational Foundations                    Marcus B. Weaver-Hightower
and Research, Grand Forks
ND, USA

REFERENCES

Gilbert, G., & Walker, D. (Directors). (2005). *Jamie's school dinners* [Television series]. London: Freemantle Media.

Goffman, E. (1962). *Asylums: Essays on the social situation of mental patients and other inmates.* Chicago: Aldine Publishing.

Kenner, R. (Writer), & Schlosser E. (Director). (2008). *Food, Inc.* [Motion picture]. United States: Participant Media.

Levine, S. (2008). *School lunch politics: The surprising history of America's favorite welfare program.* Princeton: Princeton University Press.

Pollan, M. (2006). *The omnivore's dilemma: A natural history of four meals.* New York: Penguin Books.

Poppendieck, J. (2010). *Free for all: Fixing school food in America.* Berkeley: University of California Press.

Rice, S. (Ed.) (2013). School lunch [Special issue]. *Journal of Thought, 48*(2).

Schlosser, E. (2001). *Fast food nation: The dark side of the all-American meal.* Boston: Houghton Mifflin Company.

Smith, B. (Director). (2010). *Jamie Oliver's food revolution* [television series]. New York: American Broadcasting Corporation (ABC).

Weaver-Hightower, M. B. (2011). Why educational researchers should take school food seriously. *Educational Researcher, 40*(1), 15–21. https://doi.org/10.310 2/0013189X10397043.

# CONTENTS

# NOTES ON CONTRIBUTORS

**Susan M. Bashinski** is Associate Professor of Special Education at Missouri Western State University. Her research interests include early communication and language development and augmentative and non-symbolic communication. She has numerous publications and presentations related to these topics.

**Person Cole** has worked with students of grades 1–12 in traditional and alternative schools in the areas of special education and mathematics as a public school teacher in Central Michigan for over 35 years. The last 17 years of her career she served as a teacher consultant, leading professional development in teaching and learning as well as in accessing community resources to support students.

**Shannon C. Gleason** is Assistant Professor of Multicultural Education and Social Justice at Westfield State University. Her research interests are in the foundations of education, gender and race in education policy, and poststructural theory and methodology.

**Alison Happel-Parkins** is Assistant Professor of Qualitative Methodology in the Department of Counseling, Educational Psychology, and Research at the University of Memphis. She teaches graduate-level qualitative research courses. Her research interests center around feminist theories, feminist poststructuralism in qualitative research, and social and environmental justice. Her background in women's studies, cultural anthropology, and social foundations of education inform her current research interests and projects.

**Susan Laird** is Professor of Educational Leadership and Policy Studies, also of Women's and Gender Studies and of Human Relations, at the University of Oklahoma, where she is Educational Studies program coordinator. Author of *Mary Wollstonecraft: Philosophical Mother of Coeducation* and many articles and book chapters, she is the immediate past president of the American Educational Studies Association and also a past president of the Philosophy of Education Society, the Society of Philosophy and History of Education, and the Society for Educating Women.

**Deana Leahy** is Senior Lecturer in Health Education in the Faculty of Education at Monash University, Australia. Her research interest is the critical study of health education. She draws on poststructural theories to examine questions related to health education curriculum and pedagogy.

**Matthew T. Lewis** He specialized in anthropology of education and philosophy of education. He was especially interested in urban education, which he analyzed mainly through the lens of poststructural theory. Dr. Lewis passed away in June 2017.

**John Lupinacci** is an assistant professor at the Washington State University. He teaches pre-service teachers and graduate students in the Cultural Studies and Social Thought in Education (CSSTE) program using an approach that advocates for the development of scholar-activist educators. His experiences teaching as a high school math and science teacher, an outdoor environmental educator, and a community activist all contribute to examining the relationships between schools and the reproduction of the cultural roots of social suffering and environmental degradation.

**Jennifer C. Ng** is an associate professor in the Department of Educational Leadership and Policy Studies at the University of Kansas. Her scholarly interests include examining how educators address diversity and multiculturalism in K–12 and higher education settings. Her recent work has appeared in journals such as *The Urban Review* and *Teachers College Record*.

**Carolyn Pluim** is an associate professor and Chair of the Department of Leadership, Educational Psychology, and Foundations at Northern Illinois University. Her research interests are in the foundations of education and educational policy studies. Her work specifically examines school health policies and practices and how these are enacted in schools.

**Darren Powell** is Lecturer in Health Education in the Faculty of Education and Social Work, University of Auckland. He is currently leading a research project on the impact of marketing 'health' to children. His research interests include the childhood obesity 'crisis'; children's perspectives of health, fitness, and fatness; and the corporatisation of public education.

**Suzanne Rice** is Professor of Education at the University of Kansas. Her interests include philosophy of education, food ethics, anthrozoology, and education policy. Her recent publications appeared in *Teachers College Record*, *Educational Theory*, and *Journal of Thought*.

**A. G. Rud** is a distinguished Professor of Education at Washington State University. His interests include the cultural foundations of education, with particular emphasis on the moral dimensions of teaching, learning, and leading. His recent books include *The educational significance of human and non-human animal interactions: Blurring the species line*. New York, NY: Palgrave Macmillan, co-edited with Suzanne Rice and *Teaching with reverence: Reviving an ancient virtue for today's schools*. New York, NY: Palgrave Macmillan, co-edited with Jim Garrison.

**Paula M. Salvio** is Professor of Education in the College of Liberal Arts and an Education, Culture, and Sustainability scholar in the Sustainability Institute at the University of New Hampshire. Her research focuses on the cultural and historical foundations of education, areas in which she has published widely.

**Kip Smilie** is Assistant Professor of Education at Missouri Western State University. His research interests include philosophical, historical, and social foundations of education. He has published on topics including John Dewey, Plato, the humanist curriculum, and leisure's place in education.

**Sarah R. Stapleton** is an assistant professor in the Education Studies department at the University of Oregon's College of Education. Her research interests involve critical cultural studies of science and environmental education, with an emphasis on food in and around schools.

**Marcus Weaver-Hightower** is a professor in the Department of Educational Foundations and Research at the University of North Dakota. His research focuses on food politics, masculinity studies, and the politics

xviii    NOTES ON CONTRIBUTORS

and sociology of education and policy. He is the author of numerous articles and his work has been awarded the 2013 Anselm Strauss Award for Qualitative Family Research from the National Council on Family Relations as well as a Critics Choice Book Award from the American Educational Studies Association.

# LIST OF FIGURES

CHAPTER 1

# Introduction

*Suzanne Rice and A. G. Rud*

As of fall 2016, about 50.4 million students attended public elementary and secondary schools in the United States and an additional 5.2 million attended private schools (National Center for Educational Statistics 2015). Essentially every student eats lunch during the school days, and yet this multifaceted noontime phenomenon has received less attention in the education literature than practically any other school activity. Interestingly, the most widely cited books on school lunch in the United States are written by scholars outside the broad field of education (Levine 2008; Poppendieck 2010). The relative lack of educational scholarship on food more broadly and school lunch in particular is highlighted by two groundbreaking essays.

In her 2007 Presidential Address to the Philosophy of Education Society, Susan Laird draws attention to the fact that food, a most basic human need and the "object" around which, historically, most humans' lives have been organized (and many lives are still organized today), is now rarely a topic of discussion or scholarly inquiry in education. This has not always been the case, Laird notes, recalling the works of Plato, Locke,

S. Rice (✉)
University of Kansas, Lawrence, KS, USA

A. G. Rud
Washington State University, Pullman, WA, USA

© The Author(s) 2018
S. Rice, A. G. Rud (eds.), *Educational Dimensions of School Lunch*,
https://doi.org/10.1007/978-3-319-72517-8_1

Rousseau, Wollstonecraft, and Dewey among others, who discussed food and practices related to food in educational terms. At the very least, nearly all discussed some aspects of the relation between food and students' physical and mental well-being. Most went some distance beyond that to address such topics as the educational significance of various food-related practices, such as farming, cooking, and serving, and the role of food (and eating) in the formation of attitudes, tastes, desires, and habits. Laird adopts the term "foodways," which in her account covers "what, how, with whom, when, where, how much, by what labors and whose labors, from what markets and ecosystems, and even why and with what consequences people eat and drink (or do not eat and drink)" (Laird 2008, p. 1). Given their centrality in human experience, foodways, Laird argues, should again become foci of educational inquiry.

In an article published in *Educational Researcher* three years later, Weaver-Hightower addresses *school* food in particular (2011). When most adults reflect on their experiences with school food, images of compartmentalized trays, vending machines, or a cherished lunchbox may come to mind. Perhaps memory turns to especially pleasant or painful lunchroom interactions, special treats offered around the holidays, or the aroma of fish sticks on Fridays. While among the most common, such memories concern only a small fraction of the ways in which food is presented in schools. Weaver-Hightower points out that school food is related, centrally or peripherally, to practically *every* aspect of schooling, including (but not limited to) student health, achievement, and attainment; teaching, administration, and educational politics and policy; businesses that produce and supply food and the farm environments and animals upon which they depend. Further, he argues, school food teaches children about eating and food practices, provides a window into identity and culture, and reflects understandings of and commitments to social justice. Weaver-Hightower concludes his essay much like Laird, arguing that the pervasiveness and significance of school food and the many practices making school food possible should capture the attention of education scholars.

Directly or indirectly, each chapter in this book answers Laird's and Weaver-Hightower's calls for inquiry into food and school lunch. The essays collected here are diverse in terms of their particular interests, theoretical orientations, and value commitments. What unites this eclectic collection is its central purpose: to examine school lunch as an educational phenomenon. Education is a multifaceted process, connected with every dimension of the human experience. The authors contributing to this volume are interested in how various aspects of school lunch affect the health, the intellectual, moral, and emotional development, and the overall well-being of those whose lives are affected—directly or indirectly—with this aspect of schooling. We are interested not only in the near-term educational effects of particular school lunch practices, but also in those that are long-lasting. Education, by its nature, tends to live on in each of us. Our preferences, choices, and conduct in the current moment embody traces of educational events that occurred earlier, sometimes much earlier, in our lives. To pick a familiar example, we may be unable to identify an "aha moment" when reading became second nature, but each time we encounter the written word, we are connected with educational events undergone long ago in elementary school where we learned to make sense of certain kinds of symbols. While education lives on in us as individuals, it also, in a way, stretches out beyond the individual; the effects of education are far reaching. We are accustomed to thinking about education in terms of its consequences for those most directly involved, especially students (and also sometimes parents, teachers, and administrators), but it is important to recognize that education has consequences for many other beings and entities—humans, animals, the environment, and the world as a whole.

What we eat and how we eat, and how we think about food and eating, are of course partly a result of our nature as a species, but to a very large extent, these are also a result of education. This education comes from many sources, one of which is the school. Learning *to eat* certain foods and learning *about* food and eating in school are learning that occurs in a particular social context. That social context leaves its mark on what is learned, and while much of that learning concerns food, it also concerns social relations between those who eat, the students, and beyond that, to all those who make school food possible and those who are indirectly affected by school food, which include, to some extent, pretty much everyone.

As the book's title may suggest, the chapters' authors take a critical stance toward the topics they examine, questioning and investigating often taken-for-granted assumptions that arise in relation to school lunch. Indeed, the basic premise of this book—that school lunch is an educationally significant phenomenon—developed out of a critical examination of the widespread assumption that school lunch is little more than an interruption to the actual work of schooling. But the critical orientation of the book does not manifest as mere rejection of existing ideas, policies, or approaches. While the authors are critical of the different understandings and undertakings they address, they also offer alternatives to them. These alternatives range from radically rethinking established conceptions of education and ways of engaging with food to working within existing parameters of both while making curricular and/or pedagogical changes and other adjustments in the direction of progressive reform.

Susan Laird builds upon her previous work (2008) on the educational significance of food, elaborating the metaphor "education as healthy nourishment." Central to Laird's chapter is a discussion of the educational significance of Alice Waters Edible School Yard project in Berkeley, California. Waters, a former teacher, turned her attention to a public middle school in Berkeley and transformed it into a place where food production, preparation, service, consumption, and appreciation are all central educational activities. The currently dominant educational ideology, characterized by assessment, measurement, and control, has supplanted once canonical educational thought from Pestalozzi, Froebel, Dewey, and Montessori. Waters's example reminds us of strands in this earlier thought and reframes school lunch as central rather than peripheral to schooling and its educational project. Cautioning against trendy school gardening that occurs without critique of school authoritarianism, Laird looks to Waters where we as educators can "study and take seriously the deep-rooted wisdom in her imaginative rethinking of public-school lunch as an *educational* institution that can transform taken-for-granted school cultures with its own nourishment ethos, aesthetic, ecological values, aims, curricula, pedagogies, and problems."

We have reprinted an essay by the late Matthew T. Lewis that seeks new avenues for theorizing school lunch (2013).[1] Lewis begins by exploring the school lunchroom as a site of disciplinary power. The modern lunchroom came into being in the Progressive Era but remains, in certain respects, much the same to this day. The room is nearly always square or rectangular and is designed so that bodies will move predictably through its space; it is designed and governed in such a way that disruptions to its order can be easily seen and corrected by teachers and administrators. By these and other means, the lunchroom, Lewis argues, is structured to produce obedient, docile bodies. Next Lewis explores the ontological status of food. School lunch is part of our contemporary foodscape, which is characterized above all by simulation. On Lewis's account, within this foodscape the eater is a passive spectator of simulated "Frankenfood," constrained in her ability to enact an effective revolt or to achieve alimentary freedom. Finally, reflecting his belief in the possibility that our bodies can be reclaimed and liberated, Lewis outlines a form of practice he calls "alimentary freedom." The Edible Schoolyard at Martin Luther King, Jr. Middle School (discussed by Susan Laird in this volume), is seen by Lewis as challenging the food policies he criticizes. Beyond efforts to involve students in the production and preparation of good food, Lewis believes that we need a new dietetic rooted in ethical habits of eating. Cultivating such an ethic will require fundamentally rethinking school lunch:

> With respect to lunch, then, we need to eschew nutritional guidelines and circumscribed food choices, which position the eater as object of nutritive management, and reconceptualize lunch as an educative moment. Why not teach children, first and foremost, that foods are a source of pleasure and, secondly, a pleasure that must be managed? These two simple suggestions would have the effect of transmogrifying food from an instrument to a pleasure and shifting the locus of power from external authorities to the properly educated and empowered alimentary subject.

Carolyn Pluim, Darren Powell, and Deana Leahy bring an international perspective to bear on school lunch, examining school lunch policies and practices in United States, Australia, and New Zealand. Certain of these policies and practices, they find, are animated by a desire to regulate consumption and to engender particular values, especially in respect to what constitutes healthy and unhealthy food choices. These diet-related values are embedded in an ideology the authors call "healthism," according to which health and illness are largely results of individual choices. Under this ideology, the myriad social, political, and economic factors that shape food choices and influence health recede from view. Healthism normalizes the surveillance of students' lunches and dictates that teachers monitor what students are eating. As teachers inspect and comment on students' lunches, they not only pass judgment (Good choice! Or, too much fat!), but also teach, indirectly, what counts as healthy, acceptable food. In this way, the lunchbox is revealed as a transnational strategy for "promoting and legitimizing ideological and normative messages around health, consumption and responsibility while at the same time delegitimizing others."

Paula Salvio explores relations between eating, emotional life, and democracy, and discusses how these relations have informed and continue to inform US public school lunch programs. Salvio begins by providing a historical narrative of the genesis of the American school lunch program in the 1940s, highlighting the pivotal role played by anthropologist Margaret Mead. Faced with competing needs related to human nutrition, ethical and religious diversity, and resources, Mead argued on behalf of food that was bland and broadly inoffensive: "School lunchrooms and other cafeterias, Mead believed, should offer only 'food that is fairly innocuous and has low emotional value'" (Levine 2008, p. 68). Whatever the benefits of school lunch menus informed by Mead, there were also costs. Most significantly, Salvio argues, bland, homogeneous school food failed to nurture sensitivity to or appreciation for culture-linked pleasures and perspectives.

Today, most students in the United States attending public schools, especially those in poor neighborhoods, are recipients of a school lunch legacy that includes "innocuous" food and that lacks connections with local communities that "might serve as vibrant sources of nourishment and gustatory pleasure." In place of current school lunch practice, Salvio recommends an alternative that involves community members and caters to multiple tastes. She believes that such an alternative practice "holds the promise of promoting a form of citizenship that cares about particularized others -their traditions, pleasures and appetites."

John J. Lupinacci and Alison Happel-Parkins discuss what can be learned from efforts to resist "food enclosures," which they define as "socio-political and economic arrangements that limit access to the production, preparation, and consumption of local, healthy, and culturally relevant food." In their chapter, such resistance is illustrated by the Detroit Black Community Food Security Network (DBCFSN), a learning community of food activists and producers that engages in sustainable farming projects in the city. The DBCFSN works to ensure that all children in Detroit are able to attend schools that plant, tend, and harvest food as part of the school's curriculum. The schools with which they have partnered have become sources of food and places where community members can learn to prepare and eat locally cultivated, culturally appropriate, healthy, and affordable food. This example highlights the educative potential of a "commons curriculum" that is grounded in relationships and things— such as the need for nutritious food—we share in common.

Suzanne Rice observes that most students (like the rest of us) rarely think about the food they eat beyond the food itself and are unaware of how the hamburger or chicken patty they enjoy at lunchtime is connected to the environment and climate, to other-than-human-animals used as food, and to human health—that of the student-consumer himself or herself or the workers who helped produce the food eaten. Rice is concerned that when students are unaware that the food they consume is related to phenomena and entities beyond the food itself, their capacity for engaging in the food system responsibly is significantly diminished.

Rice offers an educational response to students' obliviousness that draws on ideas developed by Phillip Phenix. Above all, Phenix saw education as a process by which the typically unremarkable is made meaningful. In his words, "It is the office of education to widen one's view of life, to deepen insight into relationships, and to counteract the provincialism of customary existence—in short to engender an integrated outlook" (Phenix 1964, pp. 3–4). In light of this conception of education, Rice explores what might be entailed in helping students gain a more "integrated outlook" in respect to food, particularly food derived from other animals, consumed as part of school lunch and throughout the day. She sees an integrated outlook as one in which connections and relations become clearer; it is an outlook in which each part of a multifaceted phenomenon is increasingly understood in terms of its bearing on one or more of the other parts and how these parts work together and comprise the whole. As students gain a more integrated outlook, they will begin to perceive connections and relations between, for example, their burger and climate change, the suffering of industrially farmed cows, or, perhaps, their own or a parent's health problem.

Susan Bashinski and Kipton Smilie draw attention to the facts that as students who receive special education services are often marginalized in actual school lunchrooms, so are they often marginalized in the literature on this noontime phenomenon:

> While a limited number of studies addressing the social consequences of school lunch include a consideration of students who receive special education services, none focuses specifically on the navigation of the lunchroom social space relative to this particular student population. Many of the complexities inhering in social components of the lunchroom would seem to be even more significant for students who receive special education services. In respect to this group of students we might ask, most basically: when do they eat, where do they eat, with whom do they eat, how do they receive their food, how do they pay, and which policies and procedures seek to influence their school lunch experience?

The school lunchroom is a place where most students can interact more freely than in the classroom, but this can be a painful arena for students on the margins, including students who receive special education services. Bashinski and Smilie see a need for further study of the lunchroom experiences of students receiving special education services, as well as of the policies that help shape those experiences. Such study, the authors believe, can help inform practice, ideally leading to the transformation of the lunchroom from an arena in which students receiving special education services often feel, and are, marginalized, into places supporting their social development.

Sarah Riggs Stapleton, a former teacher who is now a teacher educator, and Person Cole, a current teacher, draw on their experiences in classrooms to illuminate the educational challenges of students who are not able to fully engage in school because they are hungry. These are students who do not have consistent and reliable access to quality food away from school; there are millions of such students in the United States, and the existence of this kind of food insecurity is fairly widely recognized. Stapleton and Cole introduce the new concept, "*in school* food insecurity," to refer to hunger at school that is exasperated when students refuse to eat the food on offer in the school cafeteria. The authors point out that students who are already food insecure outside of school are further harmed by being served food in school that is low quality, culturally inappropriate, or unappetizing. While recognizing the importance of existing lunch programs and provisions and applauding the *Healthy, Hunger Free Kids Act of 2010*, the authors argue that high-quality, nutritious, tasty, and culturally sustaining food in schools should be seen as a right for all students.

A.G. Rud and Shannon Gleason consider how school lunch might be integrated into a school's curriculum. They draw upon the thought of John Dewey and Paulo Freire to theorize a popular education approach that would endeavor to engage students in several aspects of midday eating, encouraging students to learn about such matters as the production and consumption of food, the connection between eating and learning, and the aesthetic and social features of food and eating. The authors consider school lunch as it is experienced in three different venues: in the school cafeteria, at home (for homeschoolers), and offsite (in open campus schools). Each venue presents different opportunities and challenges to those who would integrate lunch into the curriculum. A cafeteria meal is officially sanctioned by the school, yet many students and teachers know little about the processes whereby food is presented midday for lunch.

One might think that homeschoolers have the greatest opportunity to learn about how their noontime meal is connected to wider social and economic systems, among other entities and phenomena, but the authors see little evidence that homeschooled children are helped to appreciate such connections. Meals taken outside the school or home, typically at fast food eateries, also present educational challenges because, unlike the other two, they are consumed in the absence of adult oversight or guidance.

Jennifer Ng analyzes a longstanding lunchroom practice at a small private school serving 6th–12th graders in Lawrence, KS, Bishop Seabury. She describes how, for four days of the week, students, together with teachers and staff, are seated in planned, rotating groups in the school cafeteria. (On Fridays, students sit with whomever they please.) This practice, which reflects the community-building aspect of the school's educational mission, is intended to encourage conversation, particularly among students who might not otherwise interact. The school's headmaster is explicit in his instruction to noontime diners: "One of the things we tell [students is that their job at the table], when you eat, when you're with people…it is a place for discussion. You are doing two things with your mouth at once. It is a place to share ideas, to build community." Consistent with the goal of community building, a distinguishing quality of lunch at Bishop Seabury is that students, faculty, and staff are given *time* to converse over the meal they share together.

Ng uses the term "human relations" to describe the value orientation that supports this lunchroom practice:

A "human relations" approach, as Sleeter and Grant (2009) explain, refers to efforts that encourage the interaction of individuals who might otherwise lead quite separate social existences. These separations can be caused by— and reinforced through—biases, stereotypes, and prejudices. And opportunities for meaningful interaction with others across existing group boundaries can help people overcome barriers of difference and foster empathy, respect, and a shared sense of humanity instead.

While Ng found that faculty and students alike generally support Bishop Seabury's lunchroom practice, she noted that some students express a degree of skepticism, questioning whether they would actively choose to sit with relatively unfamiliar others rather than friends. At the end of the day, however, even the skeptics appreciated having been assigned seatmates and they recognized that the seating choices made for them often turned out to be choices they wish they would have made on their own. Each of these essays helps to illuminate an aspect of the larger whole of school lunch. None is intended as the final word on its topic of central concern, but rather as an introduction to that which has, for the most part, escaped scholarly notice. Much remains to be examined, and in this respect, the collection as a whole might best be viewed as an invitation. Our hope, at least, is that readers will find in these pages reasons to think twice about school lunch.

## NOTE

1. Reprinted with permission of the *Journal of Thought*.

## REFERENCES

Laird, S. (2008). Food for coeducational thought. Presidential essay. In B. S. Stengel (Ed.), *Philosophy of education 2007* (pp. 1–14). Urbana: Philosophy of Education Society. http://ojs.ed.uiuc.edu/index.php/pes/issue/view/11.

Levine, S. (2008). *School lunch politics: The surprising history of America's favorite welfare program*. Princeton: Princeton University Press.

Lewis, M. L. (2013). Postmodern dietetic: Reclaiming the body through the practice of alimentary freedom. *Journal of Thought, 48*(2), 28–48.

National Center for Educational Statistics. (2015). *Fast facts*. Washington, DC: Institute of Education Sciences. Retrieved from https://nces.ed.gov/fastfacts/display.asp?id=372

Phenix, P. H. (1964). *Realms of meaning: A philosophy of the curriculum for general education*. New York: McGraw-Hill.

Poppendieck, J. (2010). *Free for all: Fixing school food in America*. Berkeley: University of California Press.

Sleeter, C. E., & Grant, C. A. (2009). *Making choices for multicultural education: Five approaches to race, class, and gender*. Hoboken: John Wiley & Sons.

Weaver-Hightower, M. (2011). Why educational researchers should take school food seriously. *Educational Researcher, 40*(1), 15–21.

# CHAPTER 2

# Alice Waters and the Edible Schoolyard: Rethinking School Lunch as Public Education

*Susan Laird*

## FOOD FOR EDUCATIONAL THOUGHT

"Although food is ever present," Marcus B. Weaver-Hightower observed, "its role in the life of school has been little studied by education scholars. Why should this be?" (2011, p. 15). Even while repeating that insightful question, we might wonder why should this sad fact surprise anybody? Over a decade earlier, philosopher Carolyn Korsmeyer had explained, "… if the business of preparing meals is the job of women, servants, slaves (and of course women are in all those categories), then food, the sense of taste, and gustatory appetites reside in the wrong social place to merit much notice…" (2002, loc. 789). Of course, Korsmeyer meant philosophical notice.[1] Indeed, the founder and owner of Chez Panisse restaurant in Berkeley is a woman, Alice Waters, whose creative and influential foodways have won abundant mass-media attention (Hamilton 2017). Who has ever heard of philosophical or educational scholarship on a restaurant owner? Consistently, however, media representations of Waters' talk about food and foodways reflect her strong cultural and intellectual affinity with

S. Laird (✉)
University of Oklahoma, Norman, OK, USA

© The Author(s) 2018
S. Rice, A. G. Rud (eds.), *Educational Dimensions of School Lunch*,
https://doi.org/10.1007/978-3-319-72517-8_2

11

Korsmeyer's starting philosophical assumption in *Making Sense of Taste*, an assumption that should make Waters' insight into the extent of foodways' educational significance no cause for surprise:

> that eating, food, and drink—and by extension the tastes of ingested substances—do indeed have an importance in life that invites philosophical investigation, whether one speaks of individual experiences of eating or of social patterns of behavior. ...Perhaps most obviously, eating is an activity with intense social meaning for communities large and small. A study of taste and its proper activities thus takes us into territory involving perception and cognition, symbolic function and social values. ... the values and meanings of tastes, foods, and eating are all around us and are readily revealed by reflection upon life, practices, and habits. (loc. 128)

This chapter will make no philosophical argument, but will claim that the Edible Schoolyard (henceforth ESY), Waters' signal contribution to school foodways, proceeding from just such a philosophical premise, does merit serious study by educational theorists. In *Free for All*, a 2010 social-scientific study of school food in the United States, Janet Poppendieck acknowledged the ESY that Waters founded at Martin Luther King, Jr. Middle School in Berkeley as a "high-profile" effort to fix school food at the community level (p. 225) and argued that "the time has come for a new paradigm in school food. What is required is a thorough reconsideration, not just incremental tinkering" (p. 257). Weaver-Hightower's insights into school food's consequences for health, student attainment and achievement, teaching and administration, as well as children's learning about food itself, identity and culture, the environment and animals, educational politics and policy, big business and social justice may be anomalies in the post-millennial education profession focused on high-stakes testing outcomes. But in the twentieth century's last decade, ESY—an economically and culturally diverse intergenerational and coeducational community with broad outreach—had already begun considering precisely such insights to begin constructing a thoroughly new paradigm in school foodways. Led by Waters, who values taste no less than nutrition and ecology, folks involved in the ESY project have been rethinking public-school lunch for more than 20 years in the Berkeley Unified School District and beyond. This chapter will study their *rethinking* as well as its possible contributions to our own rethinking of school lunch as an institutional site not merely of government-mandated food service, but of actual education that nourishes healthy living.

The ESY project came about through King School Principal Neil Smith's plea for Waters' partnership in 1995 and through Waters' and Smith's subsequent adventurous collaborations with a gardener, a cook, teachers, students, and parents as well, with innovative leadership from the Chez Panisse Foundation, which Waters founded in 1996. A former school teacher herself, Waters formulated ESY's starting hypothesis:

> Right there, in the middle of every school day, lies time and energy already devoted to the feeding of children. We have the power to turn that daily school lunch from an afterthought into a joyous education, a way of caring for our health, our environment, and our community. (Waters and Duane 2008, pp. 50–51)

Somehow, the education profession whose knowledge is grounded in behavioral and social sciences has forgotten that throughout modernity, philosophers and experimental educators have theorized foodways' educational significance. When philosophers of education today engage the educational wisdom of early and late modern thinkers such as Locke, Rousseau, Wollstonecraft, Nietzsche, and Foucault, rarely do they acknowledge such canonical figures' diverse reflections upon the educational significance of food, foodways, or hungers—deeply gendered reflections that offer abundant provocations to think of school lunch as more than an administrative obligation dictated by federal policy: as an ethically compelling and complex *educational* problem (Laird 2008a). Once-canonical European and American thought on education, developed directly from inventive educators' experimental practices with children, gave explicit attention to foodways also—particularly in the Swiss kindergarten tradition founded by Johann Heinrich Pestalozzi (1746–1827) and Friedrich Froebel (1782–1852), which Elizabeth Palmer Peabody (1804–1894) imported to North America. At the turn of the nineteenth to the twentieth century, Dewey taught that tradition of thought in his Department of Philosophy and Pedagogy at University of Chicago; it influenced not only him and the Chicago Laboratory School that he founded, but also many of his students and competing educational theorists. Education students and professionals today, including philosophers of education, rarely study those early modern thought traditions from which Dewey's own educational theory took shape; their insights seem to have become a cache of dead relics in the dustbin of educational history—along with parallel modern European thought developments concerning foodways in early childhood education by Rudolf Steiner and Maria Montessori. In late modernity, Poppendieck and Weaver-Hightower have made substantial and influential research contributions to the new school food movement without acknowledging this past educational thought. But Waters, whose non-academic visionary leadership of school foodways they both have acknowledged, has claimed ESY's explicit precedents in "Waldorf schools and Montessori schools, among others" (Waters 2005). ESY is an experiment in educational thought, no less than an experiment in schooling practice.

ESY has spawned the Berkeley School Lunch Initiative, whose administrative story *Lunch Matters* details (Chez Panisse Foundation 2008a). Other educational institutions are now (in June 2017) also participating variously in ESY, at 5478 locations in the United States and around the world, including 5174 garden classrooms, 819 academic classrooms, 695 kitchen classrooms, and 475 school cafeterias.[2] This well-documented, still-developing work of educational imagination captured Michelle Obama's attention, and Robert Lee Grant documented its influence on New Orleans' Green Charter School in his award-winning film *Nourishing the Kids of Katrina* (Grant 2009). Besides his film, some short online videos, and a guided tour of ESY in April 2013, my main primary sources for this case study are Waters' photographically illustrated book *Edible Schoolyard* (2008), Chez Panisse Foundation's *Ten Years of Education* (2005), and ESY's own ever-updating website at edibleschoolyard.org. Thomas McNamee's hefty 2007 biography, *Alice Waters and Chez Panisse*, documents Waters' profound indebtedness to once-canonical educational wisdom that is now seldom included in contemporary teacher or principal education and other cultural sources of inspiration. Rather than here constructing from this case a new grand narrative of educational theory to reform public schooling through entrepreneurial partnership, however, I want simply to suggest a variety of possible ways theorists of education might approach and think about school lunch after studying ESY. As climate change challenges this entire planet, could such study renew educational thought about ecological living, public childrearing, and coeducation to theorize education as healthy nourishment?

## AROUND THE PHILOSOPHICAL BLOCK TO THE EDIBLE SCHOOLYARD

Frances Moore Lappé quoted Waters in *Hope's Edge*: "Food is one central thing about human experience that can open up both our senses and our conscience to our place in the world" (2003, p. 37). Reading that book over a decade ago piqued my first curiosity about King School's reconfiguration of its playground, lunch, and academic curriculum as the Edible Schoolyard, which Lappé (quoting Waters) had titled "the delicious revolution" (Lappé and Lappé 2003, pp. 37–62). This grassroots *locavore* initiative—now an international educational reform movement inspired by the Slow Food movement, aiming "to turn the public schools into Slow Schools" (Waters 2005, p. 6)—came to interest me philosophically, amid thinking I began about three decades ago. I wondered if this creative educational experiment that Lappé had described might pose new questions about the meanings of schooling and education, or about curricular values?—just as teachers' experimentation at the University of Chicago's Laboratory School had deepened Dewey's thought about education and democracy while also enabling women's collaborative construction of home economics as a new field integral to coeducation's curricular development for sex equality (Laird 1988a). "Eco-gastronomy" is the new subject matter that ESY's "edible education" teaches, bringing together food, aesthetics, and an ethic of sustainability to celebrate "diversity, tradition, character, and what its founder, Carlo Petrini, calls 'quiet material pleasure'" (Waters 2005, p. 6). If you have read the rich documentary account of the Chicago Lab School authored by teachers Katherine Camp Mayhew and Anna Camp Edwards, who had joined Ellen Swallow Richards and others in founding home economics at the Lake Placid Conference,[3] you may remember that the Lab School's children kept a garden, experimented in a kitchen, and hosted a hospitable lunch table, studying geography, history, science, and arts all the while (Mayhew and Edwards 1936). In the wake of Unites States' dis-investment in home economics education specifically for girls and women, coeducational eco-gastronomy reconfigures such pragmatist school foodways for the present climate change era.

In the last century home economists brought arts and sciences to bear upon the study of child development, various sorts of design, textile and food sciences, nutrition, and human services. Thus, the home economics profession led the nation to see concerns about education, health, and welfare as inextricably intertwined—and therefore to care about school lunch. But the year that I became certified to teach high school, 1979, US Congress reconfigured federal government to disjoin the domain of educational policy from that of health and welfare policy. That move, fraught with philosophical problems for public education scarcely yet considered, sets the stage for such administrative tyrannies as "A Nation at Risk," "No Child Left Behind," and "Race to the Top." My doctoral research, responsive to the first of these, constituted a major prelude to my interest in ESY two decades later, amid the second and third tyrannies. For I began my dissertation *Maternal Teaching and Maternal Teachings* (Laird 1988b, pp. 33–39) by narrating a clear case of a philosophically neglected concept that I called "in loco parentis teaching": a composite autobiographical vignette about my lunchtime cafeteria duty as a high-school teacher. Anyone who has taught in a large regional public high school like mine knows that such duty may present challenges such as unhappy students who are rude to cafeteria servers and don't bus their trays; who make unhealthy food choices (despite whatever nutritional instruction health classes might offer) or, worse, have no healthy food choices available at all; who start food fights or waste or play with their food; who become racist, snobbish, heterosexist, prankish, mean, belligerent, or sick, or even have epileptic seizures; who come up to you and want to share a triumph, vent a grievance, tattle, joke, chat, or get advice. My school colleagues found such pacing-back-and-forth duty generally dull and irksome and, like most analytic philosophers of education back then, did not regard it as "real" teaching, which only happened in the classroom or library, of course. Forbidden to sit at table with students, I found this cafeteria duty often irksome too, but mainly because I did regard it as real teaching and felt frustrated by the way my school (like most public schools) framed all such in loco parentis duties, required from all teachers, as demands more for *policing* children's behavior than for *teaching* them to live well—an important conceptual distinction. I perceived school lunch's educational possibilities for the latter purpose were being squandered foolishly.

By demonstrating that moral childrearing at home has involved teaching often conceptually distinct from teaching in analytic philosophers' standard sense, I wanted to invite thoughtful mothers' and teachers' generally silenced voices into consequential public conversations about education, to invite new critical and imaginative inquiry on childrearing at school and elsewhere beyond the nuclear-family enclosure. My dissertation named such childrearing "maternal teaching," but later I called it "teaching in a different sense" (Laird 1994), and eventually I integrated it into my theorizing of "befriending as an educational life-practice" (Laird 2003, 2004, 2010). My primary sources for all this conceptual construction were novels by culturally diverse teachers and mothers who, at a time when women were not yet warmly welcomed into academic philosophy of education, formed their own nonetheless serious educational thought carefully, into fictional art—Louisa May Alcott's *Little Women* (1869/2005), Ntozake Shange's *Betsey Brown* (1985), Sapphire's *Push* (1997). I found that in all those autobiographically inspired literary narratives of childrearing, foodways figured prominently in learning—offering what in *Making Sense of Taste* Korsmeyer studied philosophically as "narratives of eating" (Korsmeyer 2002), although some of these were also narratives of gardening, cooking, cleaning up, and fasting (Laird 1988b, 1989, 1994). From my reading of those women's fictions for girls coming of age to womanhood—through the critical lens of Audre Lorde's "Man Child: A Black Lesbian Feminist's Response" (Lorde 1984)—I mapped a concept of educational achievement that constituted an aim for *children's growing capacities and responsibility for learning to love and to survive despite their troubles, especially their mothers' absence* (Laird 1988b). Although interpreted quite differently in practice for vastly different cultural contexts, that educational aim might be considered somehow tacitly normative for moral childrearing practices of variously embodied and situated parents, teachers, and other caregiving adults. My later, post-maternal revision of that initial conceptual formulation grew to encompass an educational achievement of young people's growing capacities and responsibility for learning to love themselves and diverse others (including the non-human natural world), to survive and to thrive despite their troubles, especially their mothers' absence. In Lappé's very brief early account, ESY impressed me as a possible non-fictional clear case of *public-school* childrearing practice toward such a basic, but complex coeducational end. For example, one teacher quoted by Lappé explains that "Emotionally, many of these kids have shut down so much," but he says, "Out here they can be themselves. They can make noise. You should hear one of the girls—she just perfected a haunting dove's call" (Lappé and Lappé 2003, p. 44).

Mary Wollstonecraft had theorized in *A Vindication of the Rights of Woman* that public-financed universal day-schooling should be something like ESY's, neither sedentary nor loveless, and should "confound the sex distinction" by offering girls education through freely active physical life in the natural world and mutual friendship with boys no less than through intellectual studies (Laird 2008b, 2014). Photographs and videos documenting ESY's life all seem to suggest a deliberately egalitarian sensitivity to gender that its narratives never mention explicitly, although this anecdote from Waters might imply it:

> David gave two girls a box containing parts for a new wheelbarrow. He just handed them a wrench and a screwdriver and left them alone to assemble the thing. The girls did a fine job and David didn't think much of it, but at the end of the term, the two girls told him it was a highlight of their year. They said that nobody had ever trusted them to do something like that. (Waters and Duane 2008, p. 29)

Having interpreted Wollstonecraft's normative conception of "republican coeducation" as a constructive critical response to "monarchist miseducation" (Laird 2008b, 2014), I argued that Alcott's post-Revolutionary *Little Men* (1870/2005) and *Jo's Boys* (1888/2005) had imparted vivid fictional-narrative form to Wollstonecraftian coeducation. For example, Alcott's narrator Jo March Bhaer says, "Dear me, if men and women would only trust, understand, and help one another as my children do, what a capital place the world would be!" (Alcott 1870/2005, p. 798). Waters' stories of ESY reflect an educational disposition akin to Alcott's, as she tells Lappé, "This project has proven to me children are the leaders. The only thing holding them back is adult preconceptions about what they can and will do" (Lappé and Lappé 2003, p. 45). Reading even this brief account of ESY through Wollstonecraft's and Alcott's lenses, I saw the possibility of rethinking the thin, misleading contemporary concept of coeducation and its childrearing practices in response to global-corporatist miseducation, specifically for this era of climate change.

Embarking upon that inquiry, I noted that deeply gendered and racialized foodways had figured prominently in coeducational learning at Plumfield, the "home-like school" whose life Alcott's novels depicted.[4] Global-corporatist interests that Lappé critiques dominate such foodways now, whereas ESY educates children, their parents, and teachers about the value of locally grown foods like those Alcott took for granted. I also noted that before US Congress enacted *Title IX of the Education Amendments of 1972*, home economics (still significant in African and African American educational cultures) had figured prominently in US coeducation's curricular development, sex-segregated as ESY is not. Therefore, I began my new effort by surveying specifically the new multidisciplinary critical scholarship on food and foodways that informs much of ESY's revolutionary work; I examined early and late modern philosophers' thought on food, education, and gender as well as contemporary popular works of food-cultural politics; I argued that we should reclaim foodways as objects of philosophical-educational study and thus rethink multicultural coeducation. Toward those ends, in "Food for Coeducational Thought" I recommended future study of ESY (Laird 2008a).

The following year Waters published her own book, explaining her own thought and documenting its practical development at Berkeley's King School (Waters and Duane 2008). Then, in 2012, Suzanne Rice organized an intergenerational study group on moral dimensions of school lunch—whose topically diverse work she included in the special issue of

*Journal of Thought* which she edited a year later. Rice led also by providing historical context for our group's studies, engaging our attention to Susan Levine's *School Lunch Politics*, which narrates how "children's meals have always served up more than nutrition" by serving also "the priorities of agricultural and commercial food interests, both of which carried more weight in the halls of Congress than did advocates for children's health" (Levine 2008, loc. 171). According to Levine, therefore, two sets of major players have made US school lunch politics into a struggle over the competing interests of corporatist agribusiness on one hand and children's healthy nourishment on the other, with farm-bloc legislators and US Department of Agriculture officials advancing the former and nutrition reformers, mainly women, who were health, education, and welfare professionals leading the latter struggle "to translate nutrition science into public policy" (Levine 2008, loc. 202). Small wonder that in the wake of home economics' dissolution and education's federal divorce from health and welfare, obesity has become a major national concern, counter-intuitively but oppressively often linked to hunger. Against such national maladies (Pringle 2013), ESY's core mission, according to Waters, is "to awaken every American child's senses toward a new relationship with food, one in which deliciousness comes first and good health and well being are the happy result" (Waters and Duane 2008, p. 38). Does that mission not reflect the educational aim of childrearing that I theorized as a doctoral candidate—learning to love and survive? Could philosophical studies of ESY in this corporatist era of climate change and community engagement through commercial partnerships help us to reimagine the public childrearing and intercultural-coeducational possibilities of school lunch, and thereby offer some pragmatic wisdom to reconfigure US public schooling as a strategic site of educational nourishment?

## FROM BERKELEY'S KING SCHOOL TO THE EDIBLE SCHOOLYARD

Waters is not an academic philosopher, and I do not know if her undergraduate studies of French Culture, taken both at University of California-Berkeley and at University of Paris, which led her to pursue her life's work in gastronomy, included the existentialist philosophical writings of Simone Weil, or not. But Waters' account of how she came to work with King School via ESY appears to reflect a deontological ethic of nourishment akin to that which Weil theorized in *The Need for Roots* (1943/1952).

In this moral prospectus for French repatriation after the Nazi Occupation, written while Weil herself was starving to death, literally, Weil expresses well the motive avowedly behind Waters' creative collaborations with King School:

> Thousands of years ago, the Egyptians believed that no soul could justify itself after death unless it could say: 'I have never let anyone suffer from hunger.'... To no matter whom the question may be put in general terms, nobody is of the opinion that any man is innocent if, possessing food himself in abundance and finding someone on his doorstep three parts dead from hunger, he brushes past without giving him anything. (Weil 1943, p. 6)

Weil's moral theory of "uprootedness" conceives hunger as a demoralized condition that starves both bodies and souls, for whom beauty is one vital "food" that cultivates "roots," because it addresses "our thirst for good" (Weil 1952, p. 11). Conceiving "rights" as a notion that enjoins us to honor moral obligations posed by such human hunger and thirst—human needs—she regards collectivity as having no personhood itself, but as a necessary vehicle for nourishing persons. On her view, a collectivity that devours its own souls or fails to nourish them is dead. (Ergo, an educational collectivity that does not nourish its soul is dead.) As a woman whose own life's work in the restaurant business had been to provide "food in abundance," Waters testified poignantly concerning her own encounter with the all-too-familiar urban public school that exemplifies precisely this collective condition of uprootedness and soul-starvation:

> Every day, when I drive between my restaurant and my home in Berkeley, I pass by a school. The sign on the wall says Martin Luther King Jr. Middle School, and I will never forget how neglected the place looked when I first took notice fifteen years ago. The city of Berkeley has a great university, but its public schools rank among the poorest in the United States... The school looked so poorly tended, I wondered if it might not be abandoned. Then I learned that nearly 1000 middle-school children were enrolled there in grades six, seven, and eight. The school was also a center for teaching English as a Second Language, so it drew recent immigrants from all over the city, and more than twenty languages were spoken on campus, by children of every imaginable background. The state of the school made me wonder how those kids could possibly thrive in such an environment, and what message it sent about our culture's priorities. I began to think about my own teaching years and the faith I'd always had in public schooling,

which I consider the last truly democratic institution in American life.... The cafeteria had been closed for years because the school's population had doubled and the facility was too small. The only food the children could buy on campus came from a prefabricated building about the size of a shipping container. Parked in the middle of the asphalt, this building sold soda pop to the children during their recess and lunch hour, and it also sold something called a 'walking taco,' which is as perfect a symbol of a broken culture as I can imagine. Opening a plastic bag of mass-produced corn chips, the food workers would simply pour in a kind of beef-and-tomato slurry from a can. The kids would then walk away, eating on their own with no connection to one another. It seemed such a terrible waste—all that time and energy in a child's day, when hunger might be harnessed to open minds. (Waters and Duane 2008, pp. 7 and 11)

In 1995, Waters did not just continue passing by King School: She responded to the hunger in children's bodies and souls that she discerned in that public middle school's squalid uprootedness, by blurting out to a local journalist her feeling that the King School looked "like nobody cares about it. Everything wrong with our world is bound up in that place and in the way we treat children" (Waters and Duane 2008, p. 10). The newspaper article quoting her prompted King School's principal (its fourth principal in two years) to solicit her help. Her response to Neil Smith's plea was an immense, ongoing collaborative project with and for that school,[5] which has changed the school's moral and aesthetic culture radically, as abundant photographs document this public school's profuse expression of a core value theorized by Weil as a kind of nourishment, not typically present in public-school *cultures*: "Beauty is not a luxury; it is a means of lifting the human spirit and of giving richness to everyday life" (Waters and Duane 2008, p. 15). For as Waters explains, the students "get to pick a place in the garden to call their own, a place to sit alone to do their required journal writing—a practice that shows us, again and again, in their own beautiful voices, how porous children are to the natural world" (Waters and Duane 2008, p. 36).

ESY has also posed problems of landscape and kitchen design, in which design professionals solving them have engaged and learned from children's own imaginations. ESY involves schools and children in environmental studies and environmental relations, but with its explicit aesthetic-educational aims, it is more than an ecological literacy project— even though the Center for Ecoliteracy's research has assessed it a successful one.[6] It involves a school garden, but in its moral response to a public school's squalor, it is not just what Dilafruz Williams and Jonathan Brown have called a "learning garden" for "sustainability education" (Williams and Brown 2012)—though I doubt they would deny that designation to this garden. It involves a school kitchen, but it is not just a "home-ec" cooking and nutrition classroom—though learning to cook and nourish well do occur there, where it's posted clearly there's "NO ROOM FOR HOMOPHOBIA"—for much else occurs there also, including spontaneously joyful piano-playing and singing. It involves the school lunch table, but it is not just your ordinary ascetic public-school cafeteria—even though students do lunch there often—since it is alive with fresh flowers from the garden, adorned with table-cloths, and founded on Waters' "belief in the power of the table to bring people together and give them a place to commune" (Waters and Duane 2008, p. 33). ESY's website peddles a book called *Making Mathematics Delicious*, and Waters reports that "The humanities teachers have grown to love using the kitchen to enrich their classes, and they've become expert at making connections between food and scholarship" (Waters and Duane 2008, p. 37). Within a public school, ESY has become an institutional structure of community engagement designed to offer what its founding partners have named "edible education,"[7] a concept for which they have formulated five explicit definitive principles:

1. Food is an academic subject.
2. School provides lunch for every child.
3. Schools support farms.
4. Children learn by doing.
5. Beauty is a language.

Edible education has made school lunch into far more than the meal itself: the focus of public-school culture's deep moral and aesthetic transformation. Despite Waters' conceptual and practical ingenuity in her work with the King School collectivity, I am not claiming that either Waters or that collectivity is a "philosopher of education." However, ESY does evidence creative use of Waters' deep theoretical understandings of both education and eco-gastronomy; and its generative significance for public education is at once pragmatic, variegated, and complex, worthy of both empirical investigations and philosophical inquiries of various sorts. Meanwhile, the present global context imposes ever more urgent local challenges upon us—tornadoes, dust storms, droughts, heat-waves, wildfires, hurricanes, floods, lethal leaks of oil and radiation and methane, famines, lead-poisoned water—whose violence deepens social inequalities.

The foundations of earthly life itself, everything we do to feed, shelter, nurture, and heal ourselves and future generations, must become open to question—and to learning whose necessity few contemporary education professionals have even acknowledged yet, much less tried to imagine (Laird 2017, 2013a, b, p. 132). Against that perilous professional indifference, ESY is focusing young students and their educators precisely on that necessary thoughtful practical effort of intercultural-coeducational childrearing in public schools, with a view toward preserving students' lives from both environmental and social harms, fostering their growth in ways that sustain both environmental and human health, and educating them to develop nature-loving life-practices (Laird 2017). Could further studies of this "rethinking school lunch" project focus philosophers of education on that complex effort too?

## From Casa dei Bambini to the Edible Schoolyard

Over three decades ago, in "Excluding Women from the Educational Realm," Jane Roland Martin pointed out that Maria Montessori was the only woman whose educational thought Robert Ulich had included in his heavy tome, *Three Thousand Years of Educational Wisdom* (Martin 1982/1994; Ulich 1947), and since then, Alice Waters, who studied at the International Montessori Institute in London, has claimed Montessori's strong, direct influence on her own conception of ESY. Indeed, although Berkeley's King School is not reducible to its ESY—for it has always been subject to state regulation, "No Child Left Behind" and most recently "Race to the Top"—*Dr. Montessori's Own Handbook*'s description of *Casa dei Bambini* does resemble King School's ESY as I found it on tour:

> The "Children's House" is the *environment* which is offered to the child that he may be given the opportunity of developing his activities. This kind of school is not of a fixed type, but may vary according to the financial resources at disposal and to the opportunities afforded by the environment. It ought to be … a set of rooms with a garden of which the children are the masters. A garden which contains shelters is ideal, because the children can play or sleep under them, and can also bring their tables out to work or dine. In this way they may live almost entirely in the open air, and are protected at the same time from rain and sun. (Montessori 1914, pp. 11–12)

Montessori conceived her *Casa dei Bambini* in response to children living in the demoralizing, miseducative squalor of an urban tenement district,

Rome's San Lorenzo Quarter, whose horrors she describes at some length, much as Waters has described those at Berkeley's King School before its transformation by ESY. The resemblance between Montessori's motive and Waters' motive could hardly be clearer; it is evident also in Grant's 2009 film, *Nourishing the Kids of Katrina*. Waters has read in the subtlety of Montessori's thinking a profound educational foundation for the food revolution she has led here. The project's public documents evidence its indebtedness especially to the notion that teaching should be indirect, chiefly accomplished through design of an environment in which educative sensory encounters may occur, as *Dr. Montessori's Own Handbook* describes what ESY narratives show:

> The instructions of the teacher consist then merely in a hint, a touch— even enough to give a start to the child. The rest develops of itself. The children learn from one another and throw themselves into the work with enthusiasm and delight. This atmosphere of quiet activity develops a fellow-feeling, an attitude of mutual aid, and most wonderful of all, an intelligent interest on the part of the older children in the progress of their little companions. It is enough just to set a child in these peaceful surroundings for him to feel perfectly at home. (Montessori 1914, p. 22)

ESY has involved children's parents and extended families and other community residents integrally from the start. Constructing "the first step toward socialization of the [home]" by deliberately "communizing a 'maternal function'" (Montessori 1912, pp. 65, 66, loc. 1167, 1183), Montessori conceptualized the early childhood school, collectively owned by parents, as *Casa dei Bambini*, often translated as "children's house." But she explains in *The Montessori Method*: "We Italians have elevated our word 'casa' to the almost sacred significance of the English word 'home,' the enclosed temple of domestic affection, accessible only to dear ones" (Montessori 1912, p. 57, loc. 1017). Montessori's more accurate, insistent translation of *Casa dei Bambini* as "children's home" inspired Martin to formulate her own ideal of the "schoolhome" as a gender-sensitive coeducational school that is a "moral equivalent of home" (Martin 1992). With less explicit critical mention of gender than either Montessori or Martin, Waters has applied Montessori's educational principles to a public school and has adapted key features of the infant-education practice that Montessori conceived for *Casa dei Bambini*, to form her own distinctive idea of middle-school education in Berkeley's ESY. Both Martin and

Waters have taken seriously Montessori's theorizing in *The Absorbent Mind*, where she asks, "What is the conception of education that takes life as the centre of its own function?" and then answers, "It is a conception that alters all previous ideas about education. Education must no longer be based upon a syllabus but upon the knowledge of human life" (Montessori 1949, p. 165). Martin envisioned her schoolhome's curriculum for "learning to live" via theater and newspaper activities (Martin 1992), but Waters has led the King School to claim rigorous curricular fidelity to another principle set forth in *The Montessori Method*:

> But if for physical life it is necessary to have the child exposed to the vivifying forces of nature, it is also necessary for his psychical life to place the soul of the child in contact with creation, in order that he may lay up for himself treasure from the directly educating forces of living nature. The method for arriving at this end is to set the child at agricultural labour, guiding him to the cultivation of plants and animals, and so to the intelligent contemplation of nature. (Montessori 1912, p. 124)

Waters has demonstrated that *Dr. Montessori's Own Handbook*'s claims about early childhood education may also apply to middle-school education, for example, that "gardening and manual work are a great pleasure to our children. Gardening is already well known as a feature of infant education, and it is recognized by all that plants and animals attract the children's care and attention" (Montessori 1914, p. 22). The King School's young people care for chickens inhabiting a coop at ESY and collect fresh eggs from them for their cooking in the kitchen—an easy meal that kitchen director Esther Cook taught one "boy who was plainly hungry—truly hungry, as in badly needing food"—how to prepare secretly for himself "everyday before school, without ever asking" (Waters and Duane 2008, 30). Waters explains that King School's kitchen classroom has become "somehow a part of the life of the school, in just the way a home kitchen can anchor the life of a family" (Waters and Duane 2008, p. 30). There, ESY photographs and videos show what Montessori explained: "In the work of laying the table the children are seen quite by themselves, dividing the work among themselves, carrying the plates, spoons, knives and forks, etc., and finally, sitting down at the tables where the [students] serve the hot soup" (Montessori 1914, p. 22).

Besides her deep practical and theoretical understanding of Montessori education, Waters has brought to the King School the cultural wealth of her creative work in the food service business, which David Kamp chronicled in *The United States of Arugula* (2006), highlighting the Francophile character and transformative influence of her Berkeley restaurant Chez Panisse within American food-cultural history after the educational decline of home economics. In 1971, after Waters worked at a brief school-teaching career, Montessori's conception of education as encountering the world through the senses mingled with Waters' deep delight in French food and culture to influence her own revolutionary educational approach to developing a unique restaurant, Chez Panisse, regarded by some as the best in the United States (Waters and Duane 2008: Apple, xi). In that restaurant's copiously documented history, one can see an instructive, preparatory ground for Waters' subsequent experimental idea of ESY. She founded Chez Panisse on "the Waters credo—fresh, local, seasonal, and where possible organic ingredients"—as "a restaurant about much more than food" (Waters and Duane 2008: Apple, xiii). Indeed it was a restaurant about public education both in its workplace and at its tables, founded on several other explicit principles: (1) that "How we eat can change the world" (Waters and Duane 2008: Apple, xi), (2) that "the Montessori Way—direct experience, experimentation, optimism, confidence—would be the way of her restaurant" (McNamee 2007, p. 39), which included application of "the Montessori ideal of learning-by-doing to every activity in the restaurant" (McNamee 2007, p. 60), and (3), also from Montessori, that "You learn about everything in your environment. You become familiar with it. And you begin to see what its value is" (McNamee 2007, p. 33). Taking this deliberately educational outlook as she connected with regional farmers and ranchers and developed her restaurant, Waters later also educated the public by authoring cookbooks and founding a farmers' market in Berkeley before embarking upon the ESY Project and the Yale Sustainable Food Project. Occasioned by her own daughter Fanny's matriculation at Yale, the latter effort has gathered "people around shared food, shared work, and shared inquiry," while aiming to foster "a culture that draws meaning and pleasure from the connections among people, land, and food" by managing "an organic farm on campus" and running "diverse educational programs that support exploration and academic inquiry related to food and agriculture."[8] These two educational projects resemble both her restaurant and each other in their locavore commitment, morally responsive to social-ecological concerns. But ESY reconfigures public schools' childrearing as educational nourishment, consonant with Weil's ethic and also with Montessori's discerning reflection in *The Montessori Method*:

... if we give children the means of *existence*, the struggle for it disappears, and a vigorous expansion of life takes its place. ... One might say, indeed, that to judge by appearances, a well-fed people are *better, quieter, and commit less crime* than a nation that is ill-nourished; but whoever draws from that the conclusion that to make men good it is *enough* to feed them, will be making an obvious mistake. It cannot be denied, however, that *nourishment* will be an essential factor in obtaining goodness, in the sense that it will *eliminate* all the *evil acts, and the bitterness* caused by lack of bread. Now, in our case, we are dealing with a far deeper need—the nourishment of man's inner life, and of his higher functions. The bread that we are dealing with is the bread of the spirit, and we are entering into the difficult subject of the satisfaction of man's psychic needs. (Montessori 1914, pp. 89–90, loc. 1116–1132)

## FROM THE EDIBLE SCHOOLYARD TO US PUBLIC SCHOOLS?

Montessori extended her idea of *Casa dei Bambini* throughout Italy and then to India, and it has spread around the world. Similarly, the Chez Panisse Foundation has renamed itself "The Edible Schoolyard Project," and now works with the Berkeley Unified School District to extend the King School's approach toward lunch to other local public schools (Chez Panisse Foundation 2008a, b; Waters and Duane 2008; Waters 2005), and offers also a summer Edible Schoolyard Academy that educates people to lead similar school lunch reform efforts throughout the United States and around the world. ESY bears abundant witness to the practical value of studying educational theory, toward which too many policy leaders today take a dismissive stance. At the same time, careful philosophical analysis of the kinds and consequences of the various sorts of documented encounters (Martin 2011) that produce its educational value and its educational problems could further elaborate the ESY concept constructively.[9]

Why is such theoretical inquiry on school lunch important? Without any historical roots or philosophical framework such as Waters found in her knowledge of Montessori education, without any social-ethical critique of punitive authoritarianism in the United States' school-to-prison pipeline (most of whose students qualify for free and reduced lunch) (Oklahoma State Advisory Committee to the U.S. Commission on Civil Rights 2016), without any further foundational inquiry such as I am here proposing, school gardens and kitchen classrooms could become the newest educational fad—under the urgent press of withdrawn government funding for school food along with media romanticizing Waters and ESY. Conforming to the material basics of such a fad without rethinking what they are about at ESY, how and why, educators could evade the challenges of reconfiguring education as nourishment that ESY has engaged so vigorously while extending a profoundly miseducative plantation ethos to public-school foodways—whose ethos is now often spectacularly industrial, "a site of disciplinary power, seeking to evince technologies of force that effectuate obedient and efficient eaters" (Lewis 2013, p. 29). Anyone who has witnessed the abundant authoritarianism accepted without question in many contemporary public-school lunchrooms that serve students who qualify for free and reduced lunch will have no difficulty imagining the new mistresses and overseers of students forced to work in garden and kitchen and cafeteria, the strict assignments and no-joy rules enslaving a stigmatized class of students' learning there, the disciplining walls and straight no-talk lines, the demerits and detentions and punitive child labors, or the school-to-work agenda that targets some poor high-school students for adult poverty as workers in industrial food production and food service economies. Of course, Waters has aimed to resist all that corporatist authoritarianism with ESY. Despite that aim, in the present policy environment focused upon weakening the National School Lunch Program, ESY does risk generating a brilliant national project of privilege unless educators will look beyond the media romance about it to study and take seriously the deep-rooted wisdom in her imaginative rethinking of public-school lunch as an *educational* institution that can transform taken-for-granted school cultures with its own nourishment ethos, aesthetic, ecological values, aims, curricula, pedagogies, and problems.[10]

What philosophical consequence for public education's current reconfiguration could this school-community partnership project claim if educational theorists took its radical rethinking of school lunch seriously as worthy of close critical study? How might this educational initiative become variously configured in different locations if grounded in studies also of Dewey, Pestalozzi and Froebel, Peabody and Alcott, Steiner or Shange? ESY and its network of school disciples exercising their own educational imaginations within diverse cultures and ecosystems can claim such philosophical roots in—and pose new philosophical questions for—now largely neglected traditions of educational thought on childrearing, coeducation, ethics of nourishment, educational aesthetics, ecological education, and schooling of impoverished communities. Waters makes clear that the ESY project of education for nourishment through eco-gastronomy begs for such various kinds of critical and theoretical scrutiny when she explains:

What we are calling for is a revolution in public education—the Delicious Revolution. When the hearts and minds of our children are captured by a school lunch curriculum, enriched with experience in the garden, sustainability will become the lens through which they see the world. (Waters and Duane 2008, p. 40)

**Acknowledgments** Thanks to Suzanne Rice for inviting me to participate in the study group on "moral dimensions of school lunch" that she founded in fall 2012 and for editing a special issue of our work for the *Journal of Thought 48* (2), which included my article "Bringing Educational Thought to Public School Lunch," pp. 12–27, from which this chapter grew. Thanks also to Amy Shuffelton for inviting my guest lecture, "Reconfiguring Public Education to Nourish," which took me to the Edible Schoolyard in Berkeley, where Liza Siegler and Kyle Cornforth gave me a hospitable and informative tour of its garden and kitchen on April 30, 2013. I am grateful for indispensable assistance that Stefanie Heinrich gave me with the preparation of this manuscript and to the University of Oklahoma for supporting her work in spring 2017 as well as my research travels and sabbatical leave in 2013. Thanks also to Lawrence Baines, Scott Beck, Amy Bradshaw, Michael Brody, John Covaleskie, Bill Frick, John Green, Matthew Lewis, Brad Rowe, A.G. Rud, David Tan, and Nancy Snow, to generous audiences at the American Educational Studies Association (Seattle, November 3, 2012), Philosophy of Education Society (Portland, OR, March 16, 2013), American Educational Research Association's SIG-Philosophical Studies in Education (San Francisco, April 27, 2013), Society of Philosophy and History of Education (St. Louis, September 30, 2014), and the Values and Leadership conference of the University Council for Educational Administration's Consortium for the Study of Leadership and Ethics in Education (Pennsylvania State University, Rock Ethics Institute, October 15, 2015), for helpfully critical and otherwise instructive, encouraging responses to early work on this project, whose remaining gaps and flaws are entirely my own. My deep gratitude also to doctoral student leaders Brian Corpening, Julie Davis, and Elizabeth Wilkins in Educational Studies at the University of Oklahoma, who have taught me much about local school lunch cultures and the school-to-prison pipeline, and to students in a graduate *School and Society* seminar—Tina Bly, Lisa Kennerson Campbell, Krystal Golding-Ross, Elizabeth Kellogg, Micheal Rowley, Laura Sabetelli, Eric Sourie—whose field experiences and original theorizing of hidden curricula in urban school lunchrooms shocked us all with the urgent importance of rethinking school lunch.

## NOTES

1. Here Korsmeyer was invoking her concept of "deep gender," which refers to familiar binary oppositions that constitute higher and lesser values, assigning higher value to those ideas and actions symbolically associated with "male" and lesser value to those symbolically associated with "female."
2. http://edibleschoolyard.org/network
3. http://hearth.library.cornell.edu/h/hearth/browse/title/6060826.html
4. Elizabeth Palmer Peabody authored a documentary about Plumfield's real-life precedent, Amos Bronson Alcott's Temple School, at which she taught Louisa May Alcott and her sisters: *Record of a school, exemplifying the general principles of spiritual culture* (Boston: J. Munroe, 1835).
5. [5 min 4 sec YouTube intro: http://www.youtube.com/watch?v=qApx 7O6phWo][4 min 43 sec tour led by AW: http://www.epicurious.com/video/chef-profiles/chef-profiles-alice-waters/1915458812]
6. The Center for Ecoliteracy sponsored an evaluation of the Edible Schoolyard Project that it had funded, finding increases in students' academic achievement, especially math and science; their gains in understanding garden cycles; their improved sense of place and understanding of sustainable agriculture; as well as significant gains in ecoliteracy scores and improvements in students' choices of what to eat (http://api.ning.com/files/Hd3XFwJhO4NZ2yEroyYpmM9SWd-Hm36dOX6lIm 4NE9Lp6P0HI-XhaRvAjvohXmHteHQ7Z-9GxVylLYDN2Y-bgedbWu0IIDyq/EvaluationoftheEdibleSchoolyard.pdf)
7. http://www.youtube.com/watch?v=gD2OHk7Y_KE
8. Yale Sustainable Food Project, http://www.yale.edu/sustainablefood/
9. Here I am deliberately invoking Jane Roland Martin's reconfigured concept of education as "encounter," in her *Education Reconfigured* (2011), a useful conceptual tool for qualitative and historical research on ESY's educational contributions to the idea of the public school, now undergoing radical changes.
10. For an example of such school-leadership effort, see Patricia J. Simon, J. Taylor Tribble, William Frick, "Sustainability as a cultural meta-value for informing the ethics of school leadership: School gardening and its generative possibilities," *Journal of Authentic Leadership in Education* 4, 1 (February 2015): 1–13.

## REFERENCES

Alcott, L. M. (2005). *Louisa May Alcott: Little women, little men, Jo's boys.* New York: Library of America.

Chez Panisse Foundation. (2008a). *Lunch matters: How to feed our children better (The story of the Berkeley school lunch initiative).* Berkeley, CA: Chez Panisse Foundation.

Chez Panisse Foundation. (2008b). *What you need to know about school lunch.* Berkeley, CA: Chez Panisse Foundation.

Grant, R. L. (2009). *Nourishing the kids of Katrina: The Edible Schoolyard.* San Francisco: Nourishing the Kids Media. http://www.nourishingthekids.com/

Hamilton, D. (2017). *Alice Waters and her delicious revolution.* American Masters Film. http://pbs.org/wnet.americanmasters/alice-waters-and-her-delicious-revolution/727/

Kamp, D. (2006). *The United States of arugula: How we became a gourmet nation.* New York: Clarkson Potter.

Korsmeyer, C. (2002). *Making sense of taste: Food and philosophy.* Ithaca: Cornell University Press.

Laird, S. (1988a). Women and gender in John Dewey's philosophy of education. *Educational Theory, 38*(1), 111–129.

Laird, S. (1988b). *Maternal teaching and maternal teachings: Philosophic and literary case studies of educating.* PhD dissertation, Cornell University.

Laird, S. (1989). The concept of teaching: Betsey Brown vs. Philosophy of Education? In J. M. Giarelli (Ed.), *Philosophy of Education 1988* (pp. 32–45). Normal: Philosophy of Education Society.

Laird, S. (1994). Teaching in a different sense: Alcott's Marmee. In A. Thompson (Ed.), *Philosophy of Education 1993* (pp. 164–172). Normal: Philosophy of Education Society.

Laird, S. (2003). Befriending girls as an educational life-practice. In F. Scott fletcher (Ed.), Featured essay in *Philosophy of Education 2002* (pp. 73–81). Urbana: Philosophy of Education Society. http://ojs.ed.uiuc.edu/index.php/pes/issue/view/16

Laird, S. (2004). Gender and the construction of teaching. In K. R. Kesson & E. W. Ross (Eds.), *Defending public schools: Teaching and teacher education.* Westport: Praeger.

Laird, S. (2008a). Food for coeducational thought. In B. S. Stengel (Ed.), Presidential essay in *Philosophy of education 2007* (pp. 1–14). Urbana: Philosophy of Education Society. http://ojs.ed.uiuc.edu/index.php/pes/issue/view/11

Laird, S. (2008b/2014). *Mary Wollstonecraft: Philosophical mother of coeducation.* London: Continuum, Bloomsbury.

Laird, S. (2010). "Make new friends, but keep the old": The girl scout idea of educating girls and women. *Educating Women: The Journal of the Society for Educating Women, 1*(3). www.educatingwomen.net

Laird, S. (2013a). Bringing educational thought to public school lunch: Alice Waters and the Edible Schoolyard. *Journal of Thought, 48*(2), 12–27.

Laird, S. (2013b). An obligation to endure. *Critical Questions in Education, 4*(2), 30–45. http://education.missouristate.edu/AcadEd/75532.htm

Laird, S. (2017). Learning to live in the Anthropocene: Our children and ourselves. *Studies in Philosophy and Education, 36*(3), 265–282.

Lappé, F. M., & Lappé, A. (2003). *Hope's edge: The next diet for a small planet.* New York: Jeremy M. Tarcher.

Levine, S. (2008). *School lunch politics: The surprising history of America's favorite welfare program.* Princeton: Princeton University Press.

Lewis, M. T. (2013). Postmodern dietetic: Reclaiming the body through the practice of alimentary freedom. *Journal of Thought, 42*(2), 28–48.

Lorde, A. (1984). *Sister outsider.* Trumansburg: Crossing.

Martin, J. R. (1992). *The schoolhome: Rethinking schools for changing families.* Cambridge, MA: Harvard University Press.

Martin, J. R. (1994). Excluding women from the educational realm. In *Changing the educational landscape: Philosophy, women, and curriculum.* New York: Routledge.

Martin, J. R. (2011). *Education reconfigured: Culture, encounter, and change.* New York: Routledge.

Mayhew, K. C., & Edwards, A. C. (1936). *The Dewey School.* New York: D. Appleton-Century.

McNamee, T. (2007). *Alice Waters and Chez Panisse: The romantic, impractical, often eccentric, ultimately brilliant making of food revolution,* with foreword by R.W. Apple, Jr. New York: Penguin Books.

Montessori, M. (1912). *The Montessori method,* with introduction by Henry W. Holmes (trans: George, A. E.). New York: Frederick A. Stokes Company.

Montessori, M. (1914). *Dr. Montessori's own and book.* New York: Frederick A. Stokes Company.

Montessori, M. (1949). *The absorbent mind.* Madras: The Theosophical Publishing House.

Oklahoma State Advisory Committee to the U.S. Commission on Civil Rights. (May 2016). *Civil rights and the school-to-prison pipeline in Oklahoma.* Oklahoma City.

Poppendieck, J. (2010). *Free for all: Fixing school food in America.* Berkeley: University of California Press.

Pringle, P. (Ed.). (2013). *A place at the table: The crisis of 49 million hungry Americans and how to solve it.* New York: Public Affairs.

Sapphire. (1997). *Push.* New York: Vintage.

Shange, N. (1985). *Betsey Brown.* New York: St. Martin's.

Ulich, R. (Ed.). (1947). *Three thousand years of educational wisdom.* Cambridge, MA: Harvard University Press.

Waters, A. (2005). *Slow food, slow schools: Transforming education through a school lunch curriculum. Preface to Ten years of education: Edible Schoolyard.* Berkeley, CA: Chez Panisse Foundation.

Waters, A., & Duane, D. (2008). *Edible schoolyard: A universal idea.* San Francisco: Chronicle Books.

Weaver-Hightower, M. B. (2011). Why educational researchers should take school food seriously. In. *Educational Researcher 40*(1), 15–21. http://www.jstor.org/stable/51058190

Weil, S. (1943, 1952). *The need for roots: Prelude to a declaration of duties towards mankind*, with preface by T.S. Eliot (trans: Wills, A.). London: Routledge.

Williams, D. R., & Brown, J. D. (2012). *Learning gardens and sustainability education: Bringing life to schools and schools to life*. New York: Routledge.

CHAPTER 3

# Postmodern Dietetic: Reclaiming the Body Through the Practice of Alimentary Freedom


*Matthew T. Lewis*

The National School Lunch Program (hereafter, NSLP) is a charitable and well-intentioned program that serves low-cost or free lunches each day to more than 31 million children in over 100,000 public schools, non-profit private schools, and residential childcare institutions ("National School Lunch Program" 2011). For most children living in poverty in major US cities, it is the primary source of daily nutrition. In short, school lunch has become an immensely popular form of social welfare and a premiere poverty program in the United States (Levine 2008).

Despite its pro-social intentions, NSLP has received quite a lot of criticism as of late. Professional organizations (e.g., Physicians Committee for Responsible Medicine, American Medical Association) have suggested that school lunches consist of too many processed foods, often ignore federal caloric guidelines, and contribute to childhood obesity. Likewise, popular media have entered the fray, underscoring the ostensible arbitrariness of school lunch standards through tasty bits of lunacy that are devoured by a voracious, if perhaps bemused, public. In one case, a preschooler at West Hoke Elementary in Raeford, North Carolina, had her homemade turkey sandwich confiscated by a school official, who reported that the sandwich did not meet state dietary guidelines, at which point the

M. T. Lewis (✉)
University of Kansas, Lawrence, KS, USA

© The Author(s) 2018
S. Rice, A. G. Rud (eds.), *Educational Dimensions of School Lunch*,
https://doi.org/10.1007/978-3-319-72517-8_3

girl was made to eat the school's chicken nuggets as a suitable alternative (Burrows 2012). Even celebrity chefs have become critics, with perhaps the prime example being Jamie Oliver, who once poured ammonia on beef trimmings in order to illustrate—in, I might add, a rather erroneous way— the production of finely textured lean beef, which is commonly known under its dysphemism, "Pink Slime." ("Jamie Oliver's Food Revolution: Pink Slime," 2011). School lunch has received scholarly criticism as well, with most studies focusing on the lack of nutritious foods being served to children and the deplorable consequences for health (see, e.g., Briefel et al. 2009; Condon et al. 2009; Gordon et al. 1995).

While such critiques and studies have merit, I believe when we focus on lunch through the phenomenological prisms of nutrition and health, we limit our ability to conceptualize lunch in new ways. As such, this work will seek to problematize different dimensions of lunch and to open up new theoretical spaces for the investigation of lunch. In particular, I will explore the lunchroom as a site of disciplinary power, seeking to evince technologies of force that effectuate obedient and efficient eaters, and examine the ontological status of school food as an epiphenomenon of our spectacularized foodscape. Finally, I will sketch the contours of an ameliorant, *alimentary freedom*, a rich and variegated project of the self that borrows liberally from the Greek concept of *sophrosyne*.

## FIELDS AND TECHNOLOGIES OF POWER

Apposite to lunch we have many imbricated fields of power. We have, for example, a field of governmentality, which is a broad space of organizing practices that reveals itself, for example, in a rationalized school framework. Then, too, we have disciplining practices—those repetitive exercises that shape and normalize the body, mind, and soul of the subject. We even have a space for technologies of the self, those self-directed operations that enable the individual to engage in sundry sorts of self-transformations. In the present essay, I will concentrate primarily on the first two fields and the intentional deployment into them of ramified articulations of force—that is, *technologies of power*—those strategic interventions "which determine the conduct of individuals and submit them to certain ends or domination" and effect an "objectivizing of the subject" (Foucault 1988, p. 18). In this first section, I will attempt to unravel and denude these technologies, beginning in the field of governmentality.

Guillaume de La Perrière, whose *Miroire Politique* was one of the earliest texts on the art of governing, offered the following definition: "government is the right disposition of things, arranged so as to lead to a convenient end" (as cited in Foucault 2000, p. 208). Government, then, is not primarily concerned with managing territory but rather with governing things, where things, as Foucault has clarified, are likely to connote a complex of things and people. One does not govern territory, according to La Perrière, but rather *things*—that is, "men in their relations, their links, their imbrication with those things that are wealth, resources, means of subsistence" (Foucault 2000, pp. 208–209). One governs households, economies, schools, and children. As will become clear in a later section on disciplinary power, the *convenient end* of which La Perrière has written is, in our case, the obedient and efficient eating body. Before we can explore this in detail, however, we need to parse La Perrière's *right disposition of things*—that is, the *arrangement* of lunch in concrete and intellectual forms. It is in this disposition of things that we can begin to glimpse the emergence of the disciplinary project of school lunch.

School lunch is an important part of the school day and, as such, a crucial micro-apparatus of governing that functions through a rationalized *right disposition of things*—viz. architectonic specialization and systematization. This idea, which perhaps seems dubious at first blush, will not come as a surprise to those with an understanding of the history of public schooling in the United States. Indeed, we have long known the relationship between public schooling, cultural homogenization, and control. For example, the "free schools" of the early nineteenth century, under the auspices of the New York Public School Society, represented a sort of paternalistic *noblesse oblige* that "provided a vehicle for the efforts of one class to civilize another and thereby ensure that society would remain tolerable, orderly, and safe" (Katz 1971, p. 300). A few decades later, Horace Mann (1872) argued that universal education was so inextricably connected with governing that a functioning republic could not exist without it: "the establishment of a republican government," he wrote, "without well-appointed and efficient means for the universal education of the people, is the most rash and fool-hardy experiment ever tried by man" (p. 688). Then, during the progressive era of the early twentieth century, school lunch became an integral component of governing the school, a popular form of social welfare that continues to the present day (Levine 2008, p. 2). While a full genealogy is beyond the scope and purpose of this essay, I offer these historical examples merely to hint at the complex historical connection between the pragmatic life of the school and an overriding ideology of governmentality. Specific to our purposes, this connection is most readily apparent in the rationalized architectonics of lunch and the lunchroom. As such, it is necessary to explore the architectonics of lunch in some detail—both in its relations to governing and as a bridge from a generalized program of governing to the specific disciplinary technologies through which control is realized.

Beginning in the eighteenth century, the Western world began to see a centralization of architecture and design as an apparatus of government. As Foucault (2000) has remarked, "from the eighteen century on, every discussion of politics as the art of government of men necessarily includes a chapter or a series of chapters on urbanism, on collective facilities, on hygiene, and on private architecture" (p. 350). Foucault's analysis finds a compelling analogue in school design from the mid-nineteenth century on. Indeed, as Baughn (2012) has shown, writings from this period evince a concern with scientific planning, standardization, and hygiene, which she has defined as "a broad term encompassing all aspects of the school's physical environment" (p. 44). In other words, during this period of time we find a proliferation of discourses concerning school design, architectonics, and power. An early example was Henry Barnard's *School Architecture*, which evinced an emerging emphasis on how a problematic of control might be answered via architectonic specialization and standardization combined with hierarchical observation. To wit, Barnard (1850) warned of the pernicious consequences of poorly designed school rooms and admonished that they "be so arranged as to facilitate habits of attention, take away all temptation and encouragement to violate the rules of the school on the part of any scholar, and admit of the constant and complete supervision of the whole school by the teacher" (p. 54). At the turn of the twentieth century, discourses began to focus more specifically on instrumentality and a scientific regulation of the body. The American educationalist and civic leader William George Bruce (1906) authored an authoritative text underscoring the importance of designing a school according to the mandates of economy and utility of space. His account was thorough, his prescriptions catholic—from the placement of water fountains to the dimensions of the classrooms, the proper number of rows, and the best colors for walls. And then, in 1921, John Donovan published a tome of some 700 pages, which has come to be known as "the bible" of school architecture (Caudill 1954). Donovan's text is noteworthy because it included a description of the cafeteria, provided by William R. Adams, an engineer of hotel equipment. One of Adams's (Donovan 1921) directives for the lunchroom was that "the plant must be efficient; there must be no loss of labor, food, or fuel" (p. 513). He admonished that the cafeteria must be "rectangle or square" with access to serving counters regulated "by means of traffic aisles, leading directly from the entrance door, past the food, to the checker's station" (p. 513). Adams went as far as to specify that the traffic aisles should be four feet in width "and should, of course, be railed off from the dining-room proper" (p. 513). In the decades following Donovan's "bible," efforts to modernize lunch would only intensify, as social reformers and nutrition scientists began to encourage Americans to "eat right" and the federal government began to subsidize school lunch in 1935 (Baughn 2012, p. 65). In the course of this project, we see the intensification and proliferation of discourses on diet—the growth of the idea that nutrition, as a field of scientific inquiry, could be employed for disciplining the body and ordering lifestyles, arenas tied to broader social reforms of the time, which emphasized efficiency and control (Levine 2008, p. 14). The body, then, has entered the curriculum—first via architectonic dictates concerned with monitoring and control, and then as a site of nutritive education. As Baughn (2012) has written, "Good nutrition and regimented exercise became keystones for health education, and broadened the original consolidated school goal of educating 'mind and hands' to 'mind, body, and hands'" (p. 65). With this pedagogical shift and the emergence of a federally subsidized lunch program in 1935, cafeterias became integral to the life of the school (Baughn 2012; Levine 2008).

This is, of course, to be expected, for progressive era politics were dominated by an unswerving belief in progress, rationalization, the apotheosis of science, and a utilization of the principles of scientific management to maximize efficiency (Callahan 1962). The acme was reached in 1947, when Congress created the NSLP and the government began to buy surplus food and send it to schools. This historical wellspring—a pastiche of architectural responses to the problematic of governing, scientific discourses regarding health and hygiene, and incunabular market-based models of food service—manifests in at least two ways in the modern school. The first, which is beyond the scope of this work, is that of a scientizing and corporatizing of lunch—a teleological process of rationalization bound up with broader neoliberal reforms that seek to widen the influence of private interests, mine previously untapped arenas of capital accumulation, and increase governmental control over the citizenry (Harvey 2005;

McChesney 1999). The second manifestation, which we need to investigate closely, involves an articulation of segmented power directly onto space and movement.

Social spaces—and the cafeteria, to be sure, is a social space—specify and encode the forms of reciprocal relations that occur therein. A space which dictates that I sit across from you is distinct from one that enables me to sit next to you; a space for one is distinct from a space for 50. As such, cafeterias (many of which, in keeping with Donovan's prescriptions, are large enclosures containerized by four walls, devoid of fenestration, traversed by traffic aisles, and populated by long, rectangular tables with stools lacking back support) are social spaces that localize and control the circulation of bodies, define the contours of movement, social discourse, and subjectivity. Stated another way, the lunchroom is a social site for a *spatialization* and *ramification* of power and, to borrow a term from Foucault (2000), a *canalization* of bodies (p. 361). The architectonics of this space is not the sole apparatus at play, but rather an impetus for the functional organization of space as an analytic unit—a disciplinary site where micro-techniques of control are chosen, refined, and articulated upon the eating body.

As Foucault (1975/1995) has demonstrated, discipline in institutionalized contexts "proceeds from the distribution of individuals in space" (p. 141). But how exactly is this effected? One technique is to enclose a space, setting it off from other areas and, thereby, ensuring it as "protected place of disciplinary monotony" (p. 141). Recall William Adams's suggestion for "the plant" where students would eat: it would be rectangle or square, set off from the school proper, with clearly defined functional spaces. Recall, too, your own experience in school lunchrooms: the repetitive exercise of receiving and consuming food, the disciplinary monotony of eating in a hermetically sealed area. It is insufficient, however, to simply cordon off a space for eating: the space must, moreover, be partitioned so each individual has a place and each place an individual. That is, locations must be specified and standardized, and then expectations must be mapped onto them. One does not eat in the line, or stand stock still in the serving area, or stand at the table. The tacit purpose here is "to know where and how to locate individuals, to set up useful communications, to interrupt others, to be able at each moment to supervise the conduct of each individual" (Foucault 1975/1995, p. 143). All this is tantamount to the articulation of power onto the space of eating—an engineering of technologies that establish a precise, analytic grid of space, and locate bodies within said grid, thus arranging a bulwark against a spontaneous, and potentially disorderly, distribution of bodies. To state it bluntly, a lunchroom must produce obedient, docile bodies.

Having enclosed and partitioned a space, a disciplinary institution must then code its space in a functional way—that is, it must define a place in such a way that it not only localizes bodies in space but also ensures their efficacy (Foucault 1975/1995, p. 144). In the present case, we find a spatial arrangement that encourages a dining experience that is quick, efficient, and relatively waste free. Think of the way the body is directed. First, it is moved through the serving line, where food is placed onto compartmentalized trays. There are no choices to slow the movement of the line; the choice of which foods will nourish the body has already been made. The space is linear and narrow to discourage dallying. Next the student is led to a spot, often assigned, along a long, rectangular table. The tables parallel one another so that the central aisles between them are of sufficient space for an onlooker to walk them—up and down—making certain that children are eating quickly and correctly. Here, then, we have clear disciplining of the body, creating a limpid grid of intelligibility—a differentiated unit of parts that can be deciphered and, if necessary, corrected quickly.

A second component of disciplinary power is the control of time and activity. First, we have the time-table—the meat and potatoes, so to speak, of the school day. The small sliver of time peeled away for lunch is one part of this table, which regulates and imposes order on the day. Moreover, the table expresses clearly the forms of work that fill its parts: it is thus a mechanism of both obedience and efficiency. It articulates, through a detailed sequence of prescriptions, a field of permissible behavior for specific slots of time. Hence we have alimentary routines and expectations for lining up, tray-carrying, eating with utensils and napkins, keeping both feet anchored to the floor, and so on. This coordination of the body with not only its gestures but also with time aggrandizes, indeed exhausts, its utility. Lunch is denuded of all auxiliary activities—a dining experience reduced to a mass feeding—and we have unadulterated time that is, for the sake of maximum efficiency, elaborated and interpolated at predetermined moments by prefigured movements. As Foucault (1975/1995) has written, "Time measured and paid must also be a time without impurities or defects; a time of quality, throughout which the body is constantly applied to its exercise" (p. 151). In short, the disciplined body—obedient and industrious—is a prerequisite for an efficient feeding. As an example of this process, take the veritable gymnastics of self (a detailed series of body maneuvers and gestures that accrete as a daily disciplinary exercise) involved in the following set of prescriptions from Head Start, detailing how a child should set her place at the lunch table:

- Child will touch only his own place setting.
- Child will place a napkin on the top plate in the stack.
- Child will place a knife, fork, and spoon on the plate on top of the napkin.
- Child will place a glass on the plate laying down.
- Child will pick up the place setting, putting his thumb inside the glass to stabilize it and move to his assigned place.
- Child will carry his place setting to his assigned seat.
- Child will set up his place setting using the table template as a guide.
- Child's glass will remain on the glass circle when not in use. ("Policy and Procedure, Family Style Dining," n.d.)

This before a bite has been taken! Admittedly, this degree of specialization and coordination is not seen in many lunchrooms. All lunchrooms, however, discipline the body through a coordination of the body, its alimentary gestures, and time.

Hierarchical observation and surveillance are the mechanisms by which the disciplinary apparatus functions. Here one finds an extremely fascinating combinatory relationship between disciplinary exercise, surveillance, and architectonic specialization. Recall that the design of the school was responsive to a need for obedience and control. That is, in its design—a large rectangular enclosure—it was an architectural response to the general problematic of what to do with a mass of congregating students. It was an architecture that made possible a series of disciplinary strategies—for example, the localizations of bodies, the articulation of power onto time—and also facilitated a gaze to maintain it. The gaze, then, individuates the mass: it seeks out and differentiates; it gathers, records, and analyzes information; it creates bodies of knowledge of eaters and eating bodies. And—this is the critical component—it offers corrective guidance for misbehavior. In the eighteenth century, the École Militaire in Paris constructed a dining room with a "raised platform for the tables of the inspectors of studies, so that they may see all the tables of the pupils of their divisions during meals" (Foucault 1975/1995, p. 173). In our day, we have mostly replaced the platform with the roving eye—the moving monitor whose gaze records and whose voice corrects:

At my school, like many schools, kids are expected to sit still and be quiet at lunch. And it's not the lunch ladies who are telling the kids to be quiet, but the teachers and administrators yelling at the kids to sit down and be quiet during lunchtime. (Wu 2011, p. 86)

This gaze, a trained eye, spots misbehavior quickly. It is an eye that normalizes and maintains the disciplinary power of the lunchroom.

We should not mistake all of this to be a deterministic process: students are not automata, and bodies do not become sites of discipline and surveillance without response. As an example, we might underscore the panic that spread throughout Europe in the eighteenth century at the shocking realization that children masturbate. Almost immediately, the body became a locus of surveillance, control, and struggle between parents and their children. This intensification of control over the body engendered a desire to control one's own body and, ultimately, galvanized a "revolt of the sexual body" (Foucault 1980, p. 57) As we have seen, the eating body, like the sexual body, is a site of surveillance and control: the eating body is spatialized, subjected to temporal constraints, coordinated, and so on, during lunchtime; children are not deemed competent to regulate the space, time, content, or sociality of eating. If the body will respond in revolt remains to be seen, but I believe we can ascertain the incunabular marks of such a revolt in present cultural apertures and contradictions. For example, Michael Pollan (2006) has underscored the American paradox concerning food and the body—that Americans are obsessed with being thin, as evidenced by the abundance of eating disorders and faddish diets, while at the same time suffering from an obesity epidemic. Forty-two percent of girls between the ages of six and nine would like to be thinner than they currently are (Collins 1991). More than one-half of teenage girls have employed self-destructive strategies (skipping meals, fasting, smoking, vomiting, taking laxatives, etc.) in the name of losing weight (Neumark-Sztainer 2005). And while the diet industry reaps annual revenues of up to 50 billion dollars (Olmsted and McFarlane 2004), 20 percent of Americans are obese (Mokdad et al. 2003). It would seem, then, that corporeal extremism and contradiction are bound up with the struggle over the eating body. In short, we are seeing the inchoate phases of the revolt of the eating body in self-induced pathologies of the flesh. In order to understand how these effects present in school contexts, we need to move beyond the eating body to a direct examination of school food.

## SPECTACULAR FOODSCAPES

The eating of school lunch, which nearly all of us have, at one time or another, experienced, is a constitutive element of our current food-scape—a foodscape defined by rupture, hybridity, contestation, irony, and, most important of all, simulation. I will argue that within this food-scape the eater has transformed from food agent to passive spectator of simulated food—the suffering invalid, stricken with gastrovertigo, sens-ing her senescence in the incessant march of Frankenfood—who is unable to manage, at our current moment, true alimentary revolt and freedom. Following an exploration of this pernicious foodscape, I will begin to theorize a liberating form of practice that I have termed *alimentary freedom*.

These arguments are anchored in the thought of radical Marxist Guy Debord, who in 1967 published a cogent screed contra the social effects of late capitalism. At a basic level, Debord argued that over-production in what he termed the "abundant economy" had transmogrified commodi-ties, separating them from their use and meaning. In Debord's view, pro-duction is tantamount to a general accretion of things without referents—a vast repository of images that are valued not for what they do or mean but for how they appear—resulting in the spectacularization of society, where the image reigns supreme. As Debord (1983) wrote, "Considered in its own terms, the spectacle *is affirmation of appearance and affirmation of all human life, namely social life, as mere appearance* [emphasis added]" (Separation Perfected section, para. 10). Let Debord's argument here not be mistaken: the spectacle is not a supplementary world mapped onto that which we take to be real; rather, it is a phenomenological simulation that has expurgated and then masqueraded as the *real world itself.* Baudrillard (1994), who has advanced a similar argument, articulated the supplanting of the real as follows:

> It is all of metaphysics that is lost. No more mirror of being and appear-ances, of the real and its concept. No more imaginary coextensivity: it is genetic miniaturization that is the dimension of simulation. The real is produced from miniaturized cells, matrices, and memory banks, models of control—and it can be reproduced an indefinite number of times from these...It is no longer anything but operational. In fact, it is no longer really the real, because no imaginary envelops it anymore. It is a hyperreal.... (p. 2)

Debord's statement was decidedly more pithy and playful: "In a world which *really is topsy-turvy*, the truth is a moment of the false" (Separation Perfected section, para. 9). Stated in distinct ways, these two writers approach a similar argument—viz. that which we had previously taken to be real (truth) has been usurped by that which we had previously taken to be unreal (false), but which we now take to be real (false-cum-truth). The real has been reconstituted.

To add a final stroke to this background, I think it is germane to underscore that within the spectacular society, the morphology of specific commodities (image-objects) has been liquefied—that is, they are prefigured as good before they reach the hands of the consumer. In that way, they are both fungible and hegemonic. So, for example, we are witnessing the ineluctable charge of technocracy: the personal computer, the iPad, the iPhone, and so on. In the words of Debord:

> The spectacle presents itself as something enormously positive, indisputable and inaccessible. It says nothing more than 'that which appears is good, that which is good  appears.' The attitude which it demands in principle is passive acceptance which in fact it already obtained by its manner of appearing without reply, by its monopoly of appearance. (Separation Perfected section, para. 12)

This "monopoly of appearance"—stemming from the autonomous economy of production—has at least three corollaries: (1) commodities, to rephrase Debord, are good because they appear and appear because they are good (the tautology here obviates easy contestation or popular resistance); (2) given their pre-interpreted form, their ubiquity, and their status as "real," they are forms of domination; and (3) given their importance to reproducing social life and maintaining control, they must be constantly monitored and regulated; thus the worker, who previously could find respite from the means of production during her off-hours, now is ensnared in forms of spectacular leisure. As such we watch corporatized movies, read books interpolated by advertisements, and even live in parallel worlds, where, in a phrase tumescent with unintended Debordian irony, "everyone you see is a *real person* and every place you visit is built by *people just like you* [emphasis added]" ("What is Second Life?" 2009). The "monopoly of appearances" and the hegemony of the spectacle find their imprimatur in two related strategies. The first is the construction of pseudo-needs and the logic of equivalency. That is, this regime relies upon directed, spectator consumption of a concatenation of surfaces; criticism and differentiation are averse to this project. Second is the death of history, a collective amnesia. Remember, the commodity is sanctioned by its pre-interpretation as good in the perpetual present—by its appearance in such a space. History, insofar as it is a veritable warehouse of alternatives, is a danger to this agenda.

So, then, if we live in a world where "Everything that was directly lived has moved away into representation" (Debord 1983, Separation Perfected section, para. 1), where images have become "murders of the real" (Baudrillard 1994, p. 5), what is the ontological status of our food? To understand, we must venture into the world of signs and recognize that the meaning of food, as well as our subjective experiences of it, has fundamentally changed. If we compare the food of a bygone era (e.g., a chicken slaughtered, prepared, and eaten on a family farm) with the commercial food of our present moment (e.g., chicken nuggets purchased from a drive-through window), we have different fields of meaning. Both, of course, are bound up in systems of signs that afford their intelligibility. That is, the chicken is nested (pun intended) within multiple signs upon which it relies in order to signify—for example, the feeding, the slaughter, and the dinner table—just as the nuggets are nested (perhaps here I should say *boxed*) within multiple signs—for example, jingles, commercials, and billboards. Despite these similarities, the subjective experience of eating these foods is distinct. One might even suggest that commercial food does not necessitate a subjective *eating* experience, albeit it certainly presupposes an experience of a sort. Subway does not rely on its food and the experience of eating it—the taste, smell, and so on. It relies on "Subway—Eat Fresh!" and Jared Fogel, who only in a world of appearances could advise us to consume a diet of processed meats and industrial vegetables in the name of health, without even a hint of irony. Ultimately, then, food is entangled in interconnected webs of equivalent signs, which, taken together, are constitutive of our foodscape. The chicken has vanished and been replaced by nuggets and arches and fun, all of which are bound together via the logic of equivalency. We inhabit a foodscape in which "the billboards and the products themselves act as equivalent and successive signs" (Baudrillard 1994, 75). Or, as writer and farmer Wendell Berry (1990/2010) has suggested, the foodscape of the industrial eater, "who does not know that eating is an agricultural act, who no longer knows or imagines the connections between eating and the land, and who is therefore necessarily passive and uncritical—in short, a victim" (p. 146).

I believe we must resist the urge to understand these issues as abstract and disconnected from our daily eating practices. Rather, I would argue that they are of great practical import and, further, that the general public is keenly aware of them. Our current foodscape is replete with examples of the spectacle and the hyperreal. The pellucid gap between appearance and reality is found, for example, in an "authentic" tortilla factory at Disney's California Adventure (Lind and Barham 2004), in specialty coffees that create new memories to supplant cultural amnesia (Roseberry 1996), and in "traditional" Chesapeake Bay crab cakes formed of pasteurized crab-meat from the far East (Paolisso 2007). The nostalgia industry suggests that we all intuit that something is amiss. As Baudrillard (1994) has succinctly stated, "When the real is no longer what it was, nostalgia assumes its full meaning" (p. 6).

The school and its lunchroom are not immune to these influences. Debord (1983) has written that, "The spectacle is the moment when the commodity has attained *the total occupation of social life* [emphasis added]" (The Commodity as Spectacle section, para. 42). Concretely, we see these changes in the lunchroom via the deployment of privatization strategies, fast-food, and national brands that have "dramatically altered the atmosphere in school lunchrooms" (Levine 2008, p. 186). These trends seem to be on the rise. To provide but a few examples, Rhode Island has relinquished all food-service duties to corporations, and the Houston Independent School District has welcomed Pizza Hut into its cafeterias (pp. 184–185). In addition, 83 percent of the food consumed in NSLP districts during the 1996–97 school year was obtained from commercial sources, with another 4 percent consisting of donated, processed commodities (Arcos et al. 1998). More recently, the following foods were among the top 50 purchased foods in NSLP districts: chips, cookie dough, ice cream, hot pockets, pop tarts, ten distinct kinds of processed meats, and tortilla chips. Only two vegetables made the list (lettuce salad mix and chopped lettuce), or three, if you count, as they do, French fries (Young et al. 2012). These figures might seem misplaced given the nature of my argument, but they afford an unassailable conclusion in support of my case—viz. that our nation's school children are eating commercialized foods, foods that are liquefied via the logic of equivalency and fungible in the broader pastiche of our current foodscape.

Let us explore the argument in greater depth via a theoretical investigation of the chicken nugget—a ubiquitous, evocative, and baleful element of school lunch. The chicken nugget, it seems, has died a double death.

First, in the abundant economy, it has become a tendril of the diffuse spectacle: it has been over-produced, severed from its former signified, transmogrified, and, ultimately, made fungible and inert. Moreover, it has died of suffocation via representation. If McDonaldization (Ritzer 1994/2008) is the force by which McDonalds exerts its productive influence in industry, then McDonaldcide is the expression of the thanatos principle inherent in the hyperreal. The interpolation of the chicken nugget into our lives is a concrete example of the valorization and passive acceptance of a pre-interpreted, equivalent thing. It is good because it appears; it appears because it is good. And thus the second death of the chicken nugget—or, if one were inclined to articulate it in this manner—its rebirth as simulacrum. The chicken nugget, of course, is both an extreme and arbitrary example, but in a spectacularized foodscape, wherein food operates via surfaces and the logic of equivalency, all foods are extreme and arbitrary. Is the packaged, Smucker's peanut-butter-and-jelly sandwich any different? What about the rib, with its particle-board assemblage and spurious grill marks? These questions could continue ad infinitum.

Perhaps the question still remains of how these processes are related to the revolts of the body with which I concluded the prior section. To state it simply, self-induced pathologies of the flesh are the predictable result of a spectacular foodscape which anticipates and obviates, though the tautological confluence of appearance and goodness, forms of revolt that would be, perhaps, more productive and lasting, and certainly less destructive. We continue to pathologize our bodies by ingesting the dead. It matters not if one runs ten miles each day or remains stationary in a chair: our bodies are moribund. And, at least for the moment, it seems as though we are unable to see beyond the current arrangement of things.

## Alimentary Freedom

Despite the critical nature of my argument, I believe we can reclaim and liberate our bodies. In the remainder of this essay, I will offer a few prescriptions for *alimentary freedom*, a project of body emancipation that subsumes many related tactical maneuvers.

First, we must acknowledge that an interruptive movement has begun. That is, there are extant practices that interrupt the micro-powers that have inhered in school eating. A personal favorite is The Edible Schoolyard program at Martin Luther King, Jr. Middle School in Berkeley, California, which contests the sort of hegemonic food policies that have been under scrutiny in this essay. In this program:

... children join their science teachers in growing and harvesting Brandywine tomatoes and golden raspberries along the way to learning about biology, ecology, and chemistry. Inside its working kitchen, a teacher might explain ancient history through the hand of grinding wheat berries into flour, and the baking of bread. And it has a communal dining table where many of our students eat the only shared meal of the day, and where the civilizing rituals of the table have become part of the larger curriculum. By the time a young girl has finished a delicious meal and returned her table scraps to the garden soil, and gone back to planting and harvesting with her science class, she is well on her way to understanding the cycle of life, from seed to table and back again—absorbing almost by osmosis the relationship between the health of our bodies, our communities, and the natural world. (Waters 2008, p. 10)

To my way of thinking this is redolent of Dewey's (1938/1997) suggestion that school experiences might follow and recapitulate the historical development of humankind. To be sure, the children taking part in the Edible Schoolyard are approximating the sort of small-scale agriculture that actuated the Neolithic revolution some 10,000 years ago. As such, they are rejuvenating a history that has been under attack by spectacular foods, reclaiming their bodies from disciplinary control, and establishing new orientations toward food and eating. Unfortunately, such programs, albeit on the rise, are still the exception rather than the rule. Nevertheless, these programs open a space for new interruptive possibilities and galvanize salutary contestations that do not pathologize the flesh. They do not, however, go far enough.

To take such projects further, I believe we need a new dietetic. In sketching the contours for this dietetic, I will draw upon several sources in the Socratic tradition, for as Foucault (1985/1990) has noted, the Greeks had an alimentary regimen that can be rightly conceptualized as "a whole art of living" (p. 101). Let there be no mistake, however, for I do not advocate simply overlaying our current foodscape with an ancient discourse on eating and drinking. Rather, I would suggest that we may use these discourses as an inspiration for actuating *alimentary freedom*.

Foucault's delineation of the Greek dietetic as an "art of living" rests on three interrelated ideas: (1) that alimentary practices were pleasures that were provided by the gods; (2) that the proper use of alimentary pleasures involved self-mastery and moderation, not submission to external taboos or prohibitions; and (3) that learning to use pleasure properly would prepare the individual for various future circumstances (in this way the dietetic was unquestionably an educative program). Let us explore each of these components, beginning with the idea that food was conceptualized as a pleasure to increase happiness.

The ancients were in agreement that bodily pleasure was a good that could lead to happiness, provided that it was used in the proper way. On this first point, Aristotle wrote, "feeling pleasure is among the things related to the soul, and there is pleasure for each person in connection with whatever he is said to be a lover of" (*Nicomachean Ethics*, I, 8). Moreover, Aristotle believed alimentary pleasures were "the first and greatest of necessities" and the "condition of life and existence" (*NE*, VII, 4). Of course, there were clear ideas for how these corporeal pleasures ought to be controlled. Indeed, both Plato and Aristotle agreed that bodily pleasures were a force that would lead to excess unless brought under the more rational parts of the soul. Aristotle could not have been more perspicuous in the following apothegm on the precarious relationship between alimentary pleasure and excess: "people are blamed, not for undergoing them [bodily pleasures], desiring them, and loving them, but rather for doing so in a certain way, namely, in excess" (*NE*, VII, 4). A critical point here is that an inability to control the natural tendency of alimentary pleasures to lean toward excess led to moral and ethical evaluations of the person. Aristotle suggested that "a person is base because he pursues that excess, but not because he pursues the necessary pleasures— for all in some ways enjoy refined foods, wines, and sex, but not all do so as they ought" (*NE*, VII, 14). Xenophon echoed these sentiments, suggesting alimentary practices were pleasurable insofar as they met the criterion of need—that is, they were consumed under conditions of hunger, not in a surfeited state (*Memorabilia*, III, 12–13). The Hippocratic tradition went even further, deriding excess as a form of oppression (*On Regimen in Acute Diseases*, IX), whereas Plato argued that pleasure in excess did not accord with virtue (*Republic*, III). Here, I would underscore a seminal point: while these prescriptions for using pleasure were promulgated by official discourses—viz. those of philosophy and medicine—they never took the form of juridical interdictions about how one should live in relation to alimentary concerns. Rather, they were a component of a broad body aesthetic that enabled the individual to constitute herself as an ethical being vis-à-vis food and drink.

What sorts of implications follow from this first part of the Greek dietetic? First, I would suggest that we must reconceptualize school lunch reform. Although many reasonable programs are having some positive impacts, most are still mired in instrumentalist ideas about how to transform school food. That is, programs advocating more vegetables and lean meats for children are fine, but they still find their raison d'être in the scientific measurement of food, in the idea that lunch is ultimately reducible to caloric intakes and purchase invoices. Instead of such approaches, why not advance a more holistic conception of food—one that will prepare students for future circumstances and dining opportunities—and encourage a more educative rendering of school lunch? Here, I can anticipate an objection. What you say is all fine and well, but what of the child who, left to her own devices, cannot control her consumptive impulses? Let us examine how the Greeks approached this dilemma before returning to this question.

The Greeks approached the problem of alimentary profligacy through the lens of *sophrosyne*, a concept that, as Dewey (1906/1960) has noted, does not translate well into English. While we typically denote it with approximations such as "temperance" or "moderation," it is more productively conceived of as "an artistic idea" that entailed "a harmonious blending of affections into a beautiful whole" (p. 130). We find this idea in many ancient texts, often in the form of a balance between competing affections and desires. Aristotle, for example, noted that "the self-restrained person is such as to do nothing, on account of the bodily pleasures, that is contrary to reason, and so too is the moderate person" (*NE*, VII, 9). A few words regarding the relationship between passion and reason are warranted, for this relationship occupied a central place in the thought of both Plato and Aristotle. To begin, the relationship was defined by an internal agonism, a tug-of-war between passion and reason. Plato made this point well when he trifurcated the soul into its appetitive, passionate, and rational parts. Aristotle, too, delineated an agonistic relationship between parts of the soul, between desires and longings (nonrational forces) and reason. In particular, he wrote that there existed in the soul a drive toward pleasure, which is "contrary to reason that opposes and blocks it," and that the self-restrained person was "obedient to the commands of reason" (*NE*, VII, 13). This agonistic relationship between the drive for pleasure and the constraining force of reason is perhaps best illustrated by the tropes the ancients used in delineating the struggle. Aristotle repeated many times that the self-strained individual was one who had "overpowered" and "conquered" the desire for excessive pleasure (*NE*, VII, 2–7). Plato's tropes regarding alimentary agonism were benevolent with respect to the moderate man, whose self-restraint freed him "to contemplate and aspire to the knowledge of the unknown, whether in past, present, or future," but trenchant with respect to the profligate individual, whose soul was "poor and insatiable" and entangled "in a fury of passions and desires" (*Rep*, IX). Indeed, Plato's truculence went farther, delineating the immoderate as a tyrant, a slave, and the truly poor. A critical point must here be brought to light, namely, that the use of pleasure through alimentary choice was not circumscribed by codified prohibition or taboo. Rather, it was realized through a bodily aesthetic constituted by self-knowledge and victory over the appetitive components of one's soul, through a combative, but elegant, balance. As Xenophon wrote:

> Everyone should watch himself throughout this life, and notice what sort of meat and drink and what form of exercise suit his constitution, and how he should regulate them in order to enjoy good health. For by such attention to yourselves you can discover better than any doctor what suits your constitution. (*Mem*, IV, 7)

Both the Hippocratic tradition and Plato agreed on this general point. The author of *On Regimen in Acute Diseases* admonished that patients should not deter from customary eating habits—that the choice to take two or three meals each day was less important than the routine that a given individual had established. Plato argued for an idiosyncratic dietetic, suggesting that guardians, above all others, should develop a "habit of body" that suited their particular needs (*Rep*, III). The Greek dietetic, then, was a stylized art of eating and existing that afforded primary authority to the eating subject. The ethical individual was one who was able to subdue the appetitive urges of his soul through reasons, thus becoming "king over himself" and "the best and...happiest" man (*Rep*, IX).

To return, then, to the prior question: *What of the immoderate child?* To begin, I believe we must introduce the twin ideas of pleasure and struggle into education. In our haste to modify and tailor all learning experiences to individual children, we are coming dangerously close to excoriating our schools of productive struggle, and indeed there are some pleasures that can only be had following prolonged struggle. Indeed, we would do well to recall the example of Aeschylus in the *Agamemnon*, and the great and lasting lesson that to learn is to struggle. With respect to lunch, we need to eschew nutritional guidelines and circumscribed food choices, which position the eater as object of nutritive management and reconceptualize lunch as an educative moment. Why not teach children, first and foremost, that foods are a source of pleasure and, second, a pleasure that must be managed? These two simple suggestions would have the effect of transmogrifying food from an instrument to a pleasure and shifting the locus of power from external authorities to the properly educated and empowered alimentary subject.

The final component of the Greek dietetic suggested that learning to use alimentary pleasure in an ethical way prepared by the individual to confront future situations. Plato, for example, recommended dietary prescription for preparing guardians:

> [A] finer sort of training will be required for our warrior athletes, who are to be like wakeful dogs, and to see and hear with the utmost keenness; amid the many changes of water and also of food, of summer heat and winter cold, which they will have to endure when on a campaign, they must not be liable to break down in health. (*Rep*, III)

Foucault (1985/1990), too, summarized the dietetic as a preparatory program:

> Regimen should not be understood as a corpus of universal and uniform rules; it was more in the nature of a manual for reacting to situations in which one might find oneself, a treatise for adjusting one's behavior to fit the circumstances. (p. 106)

As these passages suggest, the Greek dietetic was neither a body of rules nor a nutritive education, but a manner of ordering existence—an aesthetic of self that not only limned the contours of *sophrosyne*, but also prepared the individual for future life. There were, however, a few guidelines.

One guideline was that the individual should eschew luxuriating in extravagant meals. At first blush, this would seem to be an external prohibition, but in actuality it was a key component to crafting a moderate alimentary aesthetic. In the *Memorabilia*, Socrates admonished Euthydemus:

> There's another drawback, too, attaching to the habit of eating many things together. For if many dishes are not provided, one seems to go short because one misses the usual variety: whereas he who is accustomed to take one kind of meat along with one bit of bread can make the best of one dish when more are not forthcoming. (III, 14)

The point is further articulated in *The Republic*, wherein Socrates expounds on the regimen of the guardian, listing a series of foods—viz. sweet sauces, Sicilian cookery, and confectionary—as verboten to someone in his position. In short, an abstemious diet was not a dictate from above, but rather a part of crafting an art of living in relation to food, drink, and one's social position.

A second guideline was that all alimentary pleasure should be governed by the criterion of need. Aristotle addressed this criterion, arguing that "to eat random things or to drink until one is overfull is to exceed the quality that accords with nature, since the natural desire is for the satisfaction of need" (*NE*, III, 11). The *Memorabilia*, too, contains passages on the importance of need—for example, the following apothegm: "The sweetest meats, you see, if served before they are wanted, seem sour, and to those who have had enough they are positively nauseating; but even poor fare is very welcome when offered to a hungry man" (III, 11). Here I would underscore the fact that it is the body—its natural desire for food and drink—that determines when one ought to dine, rather than the external imposition of time.

The implication of this final component for school lunch is quite simple. In fact, it is more a corollary of the prior two suggestions than a suggestion in and of itself. It implies that a reconceptualization and reorganization of lunch according to *alimentary freedom* will bear fruit not only in present conduct and habits of eating but in future situations in which students find themselves. Given the foodscape students will come to occupy, this is doubtless a good thing.

## CONCLUSIONS AND FUTURE DIRECTIONS

To follow the suggestions of *alimentary freedom* would require something of seismic shift in how we organize school lunch. However, I believe it is a feasible project; indeed, as I mentioned earlier in this essay, it is a project that has already begun in some places. As a way of concluding this piece, then, allow me to recapitulate and concretize a few basic suggestions that I have offered above. To begin, I believe we need to reconstitute the semiosis of food. As we have seen, food at our present moment has acquired a spectacular ontology and been positioned in a concatenation of commodities that are pre-interpreted for the consumer—they are good because they appear, they appear because they are good. We must interrupt this tautology, wherein food is an instrument, and reformulate a program in which food is a pleasure that leads to happiness. The optimist in me believes that the mechanism for realizing this shift is education—education that begins at the earliest levels of school.

After we have reinterpreted food as a pleasure that can lead to happiness, we must facilitate the development of moderation and self-control. As I have argued, I do not believe this can result from dietary guidelines, fitness campaigns, and other well-intentioned liberal campaigns. I believe that we must honor the intelligence of the child and reintroduce the idea of struggle to education. In my estimation, children would do well to understand that their relationships with food are ultimately personal and, with the proper amount of guidance and knowledge, potentially liberating. This would, by its very nature, necessitate choices in the lunchroom—not only food and drink choices that interrupt the thingification of food, but also choices of movement (where to eat) and time (when to eat) that halt disciplinary control. It would, in other words, reintroduce the *will* into the lunchroom (James 1899/1962). In this way, we might craft a new dietetic—a form of alimentation rooted in ethical habits of eating and a freedom of the eating self.

## REFERENCES

Barnard, H. (1850). *School architecture.* New York: A.S. Barnes & Co.

Baudrillard, J. (1994). *Simulacra and simulation.* Ann Arbor: University of Michigan Press.

Baughn, J. (2012). A modern school plant: Rural consolidated schools in Mississippi, 1910–1955. *Buildings & Landscapes, 19*(1), 43–72.

Berry, W. (1990/2010). *What are people for? Essays.* Berkeley: Counterpoint.

Briefel, R., Wilson, A., & Gleason, P. (2009). Consumption of low-nutrient, energy-dense foods and beverages at school, home, and other locations among school lunch participants and nonparticipants. *Journal of the American Dietetic Association, 109*(2), 79–90.

Bruce, W. G. (1906). *School architecture: A handy manual for the use of architects and school authorities.* Milwaukee: Johnson Service Company.

Burrows, S. (2012, February 14). Preschooler's homemade lunch replaced with cafeteria "nuggets." *Carolina Journal Online.* Retrieved from http://www.carolinajournal.com/exclusives/display_exclusive.html?id=8762

Callahan, R. (1962). *Education and the cult of efficiency.* Chicago: University of Chicago Press.

Caudill, W. (1954). *Toward better school design.* New York: F.W. Dodge Corporation.

Collins, M. (1991). Body figure perceptions and preferences among pre-adolescent children. *Journal of Eating Disorders, 10*, 199–208.

Condon, E., Crepinsek, M., & Fox, M. (2009). School meals: Types of foods offered to and consumed by children at lunch and breakfast. *Journal of the American Dietetic Association, 10*(1), 67–78.

Daft, L., Arcos, A., Hallawell, A., Root, C., & Westfall, D. (1998). School food purchase study: Final report (USDA contract no. 53-3198-5-024). Alexandria.

Debord, G. (1983). *Society of the spectacle*. Detroit: Black & Red.

Dewey, J. (1906/1960). *Theory of the moral life*. New York: Holt, Rinehart, and Winston.

Dewey, J. (1938/1997). *Experience & education*. New York: Touchstone.

Donovan, J. (1921). *School architecture: Principles and practices*. New York: The Macmillan Company.

Foucault, M. (1975/1995). *Discipline and punish: The birth of the prison*. New York: Vintage Press.

Foucault, M. (1980). Body/power. In C. Gordon (Ed.), *Power/knowledge: Selected interviews & other writings, 1972–1977* (pp. 55–62). New York: Pantheon Books.

Foucault, M. (1985/1990). *The history of sexuality, Vol. 2: The uses of pleasure*. (trans: Hurley, R.). New York: Vintage Books.

Foucault, M. (1988). Technologies of the self. In L. Martin, H. Gutman, & P. Hutton (Eds.), *Technologies of the self: A seminar with Michel Foucault* (pp. 16–47). Amherst: The University of Massachusetts Press.

Foucault, M. (2000). The subject and power. In J. Faubion (Ed.), *Michel Foucault: Power* (pp. 326–348). New York: The New Press.

Gordon, A., Devaney, B., & Burghardt, J. (1995). Dietary effects of the National School Lunch Program and the School Breakfast Program. *American Journal of Clinical Nutrition, 61*(1), 221–231.

Harvey, D. (2005). *A brief history of neoliberalism*. New York: Oxford University Press.

James, W. (1899/1962). *Talks to teachers on psychology and to students on some of life's ideals*. Mineola: Dover Publications.

Jamie Oliver's Food Revolution: Pink Slime. (2011, April 12). [Video file]. Retrieved from http://www.youtube.com/watch?v=wshlnRWnf30

Katz, M. (1971). From voluntarism to bureaucracy in American education. *Sociology of Education, 44*(3), 297–332.

Levine, S. (2008). *School lunch politics: The surprising history of America's favorite welfare program*. Princeton: Princeton University Press.

Lind, D., & Barham, E. (2004). The social life of the tortilla: Food, cultural politics, and contested commodification. *Agriculture and Human Values, 21*, 47–60.

Mann, H. (1872). *Annual reports on education.* Boston: Lee and Shepard Publishers.

McChesney, R. (1999). Introduction. In N. Chomsky (Ed.), *Profit over people: Neoliberalism and the global order* (pp. 7–16). New York: Seven Stories Press.

Missouri Ozarks Community Action Head Start. (n.d.). *Policy and procedure: Food service, family style dining.* Retrieved from http://www.moca-caa.org/Forms/foodservicesop.pdf

Mokdad, A., Ford, E., Bowman, B., Dietz, W., Vinicor, F., Bales, V., & Marks, J. (2003). Prevalence of obesity, diabetes, and obesity-related health risk factors, 2001. *Journal of the American Medical Association, 289*(1), 76–79.

National School Lunch Program. (2011, October). Retrieved from http://www.fns.usda.gov/cnd/lunch/aboutlunch/nslpfactsheet.pdf

Neumark-Sztainer, D. (2005). *I'm, like, so fat.* New York: The Guilford Press.

Olmsted, M., & McFarlane, T. (2004). Body weight and body image. *BMC Women's Health, 4*(S1), S5–S13.

Paolisso, M. (2007). Taste the traditions: Crabs, crab cakes, and the Chesapeake Bay blue crab fishery. *American Anthropologist, 109,* 654–665.

Pollan, M. (2006). *The omnivore's dilemma: A natural history of four meals.* New York: Penguin Books.

Ritzer, G. (1994/2008). *The McDonaldization of society.* Thousand Oaks: Pine Forge Press.

Roseberry, W. (1996). The rise of yuppie coffees and the reimagination of class in the United States. *American Anthropologist, 98,* 762–775.

Waters, A. (2008). *Edible schoolyard: A universal idea.* San Francisco: Chronicle Books.

What is second life? (2009). Retrieved from http://secondlife.com/whatis/?lang=en-US

Wu, S. (2011). *Fed up with lunch: How one anonymous teacher revealed the truth about school lunches—And how we can change them!* San Francisco: Chronicle Books.

Young, N., Diakova, S., Earley, T., Carnagey, J., Krome, A, & Root, C. (2012). *School food purchase study-III: Final report* (USDA report no. CN-12-SFPSIII). Alexandria.

# CHAPTER 4

# Schooling Lunch: Health, Food, and the Pedagogicalization of the Lunch Box

*Carolyn Pluim, Darren Powell, and Deana Leahy*

## INTRODUCTION

*Teachers yesterday won the right to inspect pupils' lunchboxes.* (Chorley 2015)

The above quote comes from a 2015 media release detailing new government rules around school lunches in the United Kingdom (UK). The news article announces the Ministry of Education's enthusiastic decision for schools to exercise their *common law powers* to inspect students' lunches. Ostensibly, the new policy gives teachers the authority to "confiscate, keep or destroy" any items that are in violation of a school's food policy (Chorley 2015). As one might imagine there were varied reactions to the new guidelines. For some, the mandate was archetypal of an imperious 'nanny state' stunt. Others, however, believed this was a reasonable response and responsible action in light of the childhood

C. Pluim (✉)
Northern Illinois University, DeKalb, IL, USA

D. Powell
University of Auckland, Auckland, New Zealand

D. Leahy
Monash University, Clayton, VIC, Australia

© The Author(s) 2018
S. Rice, A. G. Rud (eds.), *Educational Dimensions of School Lunch*,
https://doi.org/10.1007/978-3-319-72517-8_4

obesity epidemic. Then, there were those who were just baffled. Why, for example, were cereal bars from packed lunches confiscated while school cafeterias continued to sell pizza, chocolate fudge cake, and fish fingers? Seemingly contradictory, this UK policy is just one of a growing number of transnational school practices aimed at shaping children and teachers' lunchtime experiences.

In this chapter we explore this lunchtime phenomenon. Specifically, we examine various school lunch policies and practices happening in the United States, Australia, and New Zealand. We make the argument that contemporary policies are guided by a desire to regulate and control consumption as well as to transmit particular ideological values around food and notions of what constitutes (un)healthy food choices. We further consider the cultural, sociopolitical, and economic forces that render these surveillance and regulation practices commonsensical. In seeking to understand the 'work' that food policies and programs do we turn to the term food pedagogies as a means to make sense of the many ways food is being targeted for specific ends. Flowers and Swan (2015, p. 1) state that the "term food pedagogies denotes a congeries of educational, teaching, and learning ideologies and practices carried out by a range of agencies, actors, institutions, and media which focus variously on growing, shopping, cooking, eating, and disposing of food." This approach to understanding food pedagogies necessarily shifts our gaze away from the more formal curriculum, teaching, and learning opportunities to thinking about the myriad of spaces within schools that seek to address food in some way, shape, or form. Using this as our point of departure, we want to suggest that school lunchtimes have become potent sites for the enactment of food pedagogies. In other words, school lunchtime provides "an opportunity to explicitly shape, sculpt, mobilise and work through the food choices, desires and aspirations, needs, wants and lifestyles of parents, families and children" (Pike and Leahy 2012, p. 438). While such campaigns, resources, and pedagogies are largely directed toward "doing good" (Flowers and Swan 2012, p. 532), on closer analysis we would suggest that there are some very troubling effects that are produced as a result of implementing these food pedagogies.

## GLOBAL INTEREST IN SCHOOL LUNCHES

What children consume in schools has easily become one of the most popular public health issues of our time (Pike and Leahy 2012). One of the major reasons for the intensification around school food consumption is that students consume a third of their daily energy intake at school (Lawlis et al. 2016). Along with others we contend that this global interest in school lunch reflects contemporary anxieties around obesity, consumption, and nutrition (Gibson and Dempsey 2015; Harman and Cappellini 2017; Leahy et al. 2015). Following the work of Flowers and Swan (2015) and Dolby and Rizvi (2008) we recognize that classrooms alone do not serve as a singular or primary pedagogical site for young people. Rather, as Bernstein (2001) describes we live in a "totally pedagogized society" where formal and informal institutions, texts, relations, and experiences have all become pedagogical opportunities—including lunch boxes and lunchtime. Using this as our frame and the three national contexts as our setting this chapter analyzes contemporary school 'lunching' as having pedagogical implications with important material, experiential, and symbolic dimensions.

Considering the material dimension, we attend to the lunch box and its associated contents. We particularly focus on those contents that are deemed acceptable, unacceptable, healthy, or unhealthy. We also explore the ramifications when school personnel make these determinations with a great degree of authority and certainty (Rich and Evans 2005). Second, we recognize that lunchtime has a highly experiential dimension—a time for students to interact with food, peers, and teachers, negotiate boundaries, and form identities (Nukaga 2008). Finally, our analysis considers the symbolic nature of school lunch as it is increasingly regulated through policies of surveillance and regulation. Along with others we take seriously the idea that these three dimensions of school lunching constitute an important pedagogical arena for young people attending schools. Through examination of each of these three dimensions, then, our analysis reveals a transnational strategy to use the lunch box and the lunchtime as a vehicle for promoting and legitimizing ideological and normative messages around health, consumption, and responsibility while at the same time delegitimizing others (Flowers and Swan 2011, p. 234).

## THEORY AND METHODS

Theoretically, we draw on the insights of Michel Foucault, particularly around his writings on governance and governmentality. "To govern," writes Foucault, "is to structure the possible field of action of others" (Foucault 2003, p. 138). Theories of governmentality are useful to understand how governance systems and various experts attempt to normalize, regulate, and manage the dispositions, behaviors, and desires of certain populations (Kelly 2000, p. 466). Theories of governmentality can also elucidate the methods and strategies governing systems (i.e. formal or informal school policies and practices) used to achieve certain outcomes—in this case optimizing children's health. Our interest though is not solely philosophical or theoretical in nature, rather we are concerned with examining the intelligibility of the practices at work (Dean 2002). In light of Foucault's work we can see school lunching as Pike and Leahy (2012, p. 437) have, "as an intersectional space in which an assemblage of governmental techniques and strategies, emanating from a variety different sources, converge."

We must also contextualize our examination within the "neoliberal experiment" of education policy (Peters and Marshall 1996) that continues to reshape and reform schools. Key tenets of neoliberalism: free choice, autonomy, responsibility, and consumption underpin both government education policy (e.g. implementation of charter schools) and the micro practices of schooling (e.g. lunches and lunchtime). Neoliberalism is bound up in an eclectic set of economic and sociopolitical rationalities that grant a kind of "regulated autonomy" (Peterson 1997). The logic of neoliberalism embraces the same problematics of liberalism (i.e. placing limits on the scope of government intervention by positioning citizens as rational and self-directed) but problematizes these very differently. Under liberalism, health is seen as a calculable consequence of government tactics. In contrast, a neoliberal approach to health can be considered 'strategic' as opposed to a 'naturalistic governmental intervention'. As Osborne (1997, p. 182) distinguishes:

A *liberal* government of health... does not seek to act directly upon health itself, but only indirectly, in the form of imposing techniques of security levied on the environment. A *neoliberal* government acts directly upon health by giving the ideal of a series of surrogate values, entailing a sort of constructivism of goals and targets intended to bring about strategically limited objectives.

With regard to concerns around population health, school lunches become just one "humble and mundane" (Miller and Rose 2008, p. 32) practice that makes government possible: an example of how the assemblage of rationalities, technologies, and subjectivities enable those with the "will to govern" (Li 2007) to achieve its ends. However, as Dean (2010) points out—and we will show—these attempts to govern can be unpredictable and outcomes never assured.

The findings from this study come from an international investigation of lunch policies occurring in three countries. We drew on data collected from a range of sources such as qualitative inquiry, empirical investigation, academic commentary, media stories, government and funding body reports, press releases, curricular materials, and other relevant artifacts. Our analysis of transcripts and documents attended to the existence of local narratives as these are located within national contexts and discourses on the topic. Texts were analyzed for the surfacing of themes and ideas. Specifically, the following questions guided our data collection: How is school lunch conceptualized and experienced? What groups or entities shape school lunch priorities and practices? Who or what groups stand to benefit from enacting various policies and practices? Who or what groups do not benefit from the enactment of these policies? On what empirical basis are claims around consumption and behavior made?

While our findings suggest that some common anxieties around consumption, health, and obesity may be driving the kinds of transnational policies we describe, it is important to highlight the unique context and situatedness of each case. Anthropologies have long examined the ways in which food and the ritual of consumption have culturally specific meanings that hold political, gendered, classed, and ideological implications (Counihan and Van Esterik 2012). Thus we want to be sure that we do not overlook the nation contexts in which these policies are playing out. Aside from the cultural differences, there are also significant logistical distinctions among the three countries regarding the access, oversight, and delivery of school food. We therefore begin each narrative by foregrounding the national setting in which they occur.

The first of our cases involves recent happenings in American schools in Texas and interventions aimed at shaping individual choices and institutional priorities. We then take a look at the blitz on school lunches in Australia through an examination of programs including Lunchbox Blitz where children's lunches have become the centerpiece for 'healthy' curricular interventions. Finally, we consider school lunches in New Zealand schools through an ethnographic investigation that reveals how a focus on food and fatness impacts individual children.

## Serving Up Surveillance, Shame and Blame at Lunchtime in the United States, Australia, and New Zealand

### *United States*

In the United States, school meals are highly regulated by federal government agencies. Specifically, the responsibility falls to the Food and Nutrition branch of the United States Department of Agriculture. This branch oversees a number of school food programs including the School Breakfast Program, the National School Lunch Program, the Fresh Fruit and Vegetable Program, and the Special Milk Program. These bodies establish and regulate the nutritional content of food served as well as food safety standards. The Food and Nutrition branch is also specifically responsible for reimbursing schools for their food expenditures through direct reimbursement and/or food commodity distributions. As a long-standing commitment to social welfare (Levine 2010), every child who attends a public school is able to qualify for the free and reduced meal program—a designation made based on household income cutoffs.

School lunches in the United States have long been entwined in various political, economic, and ideological skirmishes. Recent debates surround various micro-level surveillance practices implemented in schools. These initiatives come in various forms—from banning home-packed lunches or, similar to the UK example described earlier, regulating foods permitted on campus (see Gard and Pluim 2014; Eng and Hood 2011). There is also the rather dystopic example of food surveillance happening in Texas. In this instance, funds from a two million dollar Department of Agriculture grant are being used to calculate children's precise caloric lunchtime intake. According to Dr. Roberto Trevino of the San Antonio, Texas-based Social and Health Research Center, the intervention was aimed at low-income schools with high rates of obesity and was designed "to snap a picture of the food tray at the cashier... [and] when the child [went] back to the disposal window... measure the leftover." The purpose of the policy was to "cut down on childhood obesity by providing parents and school nutrition specialists with information on what types of food elementary students are eating" (Forsythe 2011). Researchers hoped that summaries of the child's weekly consumption habits would help improve home food environments as well. While a lengthy discussion of the efficacy of this intervention is beyond the scope of this paper, it should be noted that epidemiological research consistently concludes that these kind of individualistic, behavior-focused interventions have no record of long-term success (consider, e.g. school-based drug education, i.e. Rosenbaum and Hanson 1998; Mackey-Kallis and Hahn 1991). At the same time, however, it is well documented that interventions such as this can be a source of personal shame and disappointment as consumption and food get understood as an "object of guilt and a reason for self-surveillance" (Welch et al. 2012).

It may seem odd for a meal program historically designed to meet the nutritional needs of children with limited resources to require this level of surveillance and monitoring. In part this is because while the program is indeed regulated by public entities there are many spaces for commercial influence that many argue compromise the nutritional integrity of the program (Vander Schee 2004; Gard and Pluim 2014; Levine 2010). Corporate bodies have long participated in the preparation, delivery, and shaping of the program; however, their current access and influence on educational policy decisions regarding the content of school meals is unprecedented. Coca-Cola, Pizza Hut, McDonalds, Subway, Schwann Food Company, the American Frozen Food Institute, and Dole Food Co. are among the many active corporate entities actively engaged in lobbying efforts to ensure their products remain on children's plates. Therefore, it also strikes us as interesting that policy makers prefer to regulate individual children's consumption as opposed to addressing the structural problematics that have created the 'problem' under investigation in the first place.

The Texas example serves as a prime example of the desire to regulate and reform children's choices in order to mitigate an unknown, presumably risky future. Castel (1991) would describe this Texas example as part of the "new mode of surveillance" in contemporary life. Under this mode of surveillance and risk abatement, health policies and practices assume an insidious and impersonal role. As in this example, human interaction is not necessary—technological precision is the intervention of choice. The intervention also follows the work of Peterson and Lupton. Drawing on Foucauldian analysis, they write, "in order [for] subjects to be governable... life needs to be rendered into calculable form... in the form of reports, pictures, numbers charts, graphs and statistics" (Peterson and Lupton 1996, p. 15). In this way consumption analytics offer a way to objectively understand and predict the subject's decisions, preference, and desires. Doing so offers a specific kind of certainty: caloric intake can be determined, risk can be quantified, and obesity—at least theoretically—can be abated. While this particular example has limited influence (that being a few schools in Texas), what concerns us about this intervention is the whole intelligibility of the project. For us, the trouble surrounds those aspects of the project that make it commonsensical, particularly given the stated socioeconomic constraints of the population being examined. Our next two case studies further disentangle this issue.

## Australia: The Lunchtime Blitz

The contextual backdrop to school lunches in Australia and New Zealand is significant to understanding many of the lunchtime strategies that have emerged in response to the obesity epidemic. Unlike a number of other nations in the Global North such as Sweden, the United Kingdom and the United States, where there is either state provision of lunches to students from low-income families or to all students, in Australia up to 80% of students bring their lunches from home (Bell and Swinburn 2004; Sanigorski et al. 2005). Those who do not bring their lunch from home tend to purchase their lunch from an onsite canteen and for those who cannot afford to do that, they go hungry. Given the "freedom" of choice students experience during school time in Australia, we have unsurprisingly witnessed a proliferation of initiatives targeting and attempting to regulate young people's school food choice during school time (Miller and Rose 2008). For example, currently we have both national and state-based canteen guidelines that attempt to improve the nutritional quality of food that is sold at schools, while simultaneously limiting access to energy-dense nutrient-deficient foods (Lawlis et al. 2016). The canteen guidelines apply the Dietary Guidelines for Children and Adolescents in Australia and tend to utilize a traffic light system that differentiates foods into three different colors: green (everyday), amber (select carefully), and red (occasionally—though not recommended for school food services) (see, e.g. Department of Education and Early Childhood Development 2012). We have also witnessed a number of school lunch box programs that have been formally developed mostly by community health promotion organizations that aim to improve the content of school lunch boxes. From a public health perspective, regulation is considered to be essential in any attempt to curb obesity because one-third of a student's daily energy intake is consumed at school (Lawlis et al. 2016).

Given the proportion of students who bring their lunch from home, for the purposes of this chapter we are going to focus our analysis on programs (and pedagogies) that attempt to regulate school lunch boxes.

From previous research we know that school lunches have become a key target in the fight against obesity in England, Australia, New Zealand, and the United States—to name a few (see Burrows and Wright 2007; Harman and Cappellini 2017; Leahy 2009; Pike and Leahy 2012; Gard and Pluim 2014). In Australia, we now have an abundance of pedagogical resources that have been developed to help schools and teachers address the problem of school lunch boxes. Lunchbox Blitz for example is a program that evolved out of a collaborative partnership of local government, health and community agencies in a southwest Victorian region. According to their website, "the initiative is specifically directed towards improving healthy eating, oral health and the active living landscape across the region. The program is directed towards schools and also targets the habits of families" (Lunchbox Blitz n.d.). The overall aim of the program is to "improve the content of school lunch boxes by providing primary schools with engaging resources to help embed healthy eating into the school culture and curriculum" (Lunchbox Blitz n.d.). One of the key features on the website is the provision of two lesson plans and supporting resources. One lesson plan is for lower primary aged students and the other is for upper primary aged students. The lower primary students learn about what constitutes a healthy lunch, what a healthy lunch looks like, what a healthy snack looks like, how to build a healthy lunch, and how do we make our lunch healthy. The upper primary students engage with lessons on making healthy food choices, using current guidelines to plan for food choice, planning for and practicing making a healthy lunch, fostering confidence in making lunch and trying new foods, and knowing when lunch is healthy and strategies to make a healthy lunch. While the learning and behavioral intentions are clear in the learning outcomes provided in the lesson plans, there is no recognition of the other kinds of messages that are necessarily entangled throughout the various food pedagogies being advocated.

Other lunch box pedagogies too have emerged alongside web-based resources. Teachers for example are taking it upon themselves to police lunch boxes and to check in with students to see if the healthy lunch box lessons have indeed been successful. This approach, though not a part of formal policy, has been advocated at professional learning seminars with a focus on nutrition. Pike and Leahy (2012) have documented one such seminar where teachers were encouraged to fight the war on obesity by policing lunch boxes. They were told that lunchtimes provided them with a terrific opportunity to reinforce learning by highlighting the good lunch boxes by picking out particular items from a student's lunch box to showcase why the lunch box was indeed a good lunch box. Conversely, teachers were told they could provide feedback on bad lunch boxes simply by ignoring those children who had undesirable items in the lunch boxes or by expressing a 'tsk tsk' as they walked past. The combination of pride and shame provides a powerful affective constellation (Leahy 2014). And while we do not have evidence in this instance of the bodily and emotional responses of the children who are praised or shamed as a result of the policing practices, we know that the teacher is very aware of the affective potential that the strategies possess. She knows for example that the use of praise is meant to reinforce a positive behavior. For those whose lunch boxes were subjected to negative responses, the experience is explicitly designed to encourage the child to bring a better lunch box or suffer more of the same.

## New Zealand: The Case of 'Natia'

Similar to Australia, in New Zealand there is no state provision of lunches whatsoever. In fact, in 2013 the 'Feed the Kids' Bill went before parliament, a piece of legislation that, if passed, would have forced the government to provide free school lunches to families in the lowest 20% income bracket. The Bill was defeated 61–59. The erstwhile Minister for Social Development, Paula Bennett, stated that going against this legislation was "the right thing to do … we believe in parental responsibility and I stand by the decision we made" (Burrow 2015, para. 3). In short, there are three lunch options for students in New Zealand: to eat lunch that is bought and/or made by their parents, to eat lunch supplied by a 'not-for-profit' organization, or not eat lunch at all. In the following section we shed light on how neoliberalism works to converge and congeal (Leahy 2014) technologies of surveillance, judgment, and the, responsible, consuming subject.

In Darren's ethnographic research of three elementary schools in Auckland, New Zealand (see Powell 2015), there was one significant demonstration of how discourses of responsibility and choice underpinned the surveillance of children's lunches. In one class there was a 12-year-old Samoan girl called Natia (not her real name). Over the course of six months, conducting research at her school, a number of children and adults talked to Darren about Natia's health and fatness, linking this directly with her 'unhealthy' food choices, as well as her 'irresponsible' attitude to her own (and her younger brother's) health. One lunchtime, a member of the administration staff alerted Darren to Natia sharing a large bag of potato chips with her brother. The Pākehā[1] staff member expressed her disappointment with Natia's choice of lunch, adding that she 'should know better' (they had learnt about making 'healthy eating choices' in school) and that it was these types of 'bad' choices that had made Natia fat. This was not the first time adults in the school had talked to Darren about 'this generation' of children having bad eating habits, fat bodies, being lazy, and eating 'bad' food. What was different about Natia's case was that the various staff members singled out Natia as a problematic individual: an individual with 'unhealthy' conduct, attitude, and corporeality, even though there were a number of other children who were fatter, and also ate 'junk' food for lunch.

Natia's classmates also chimed in with remarks about her health, eating, and fatness, sometimes pointing her out as an example of the 'abject other'. For instance, in a conversation with Natia's classmates—Mary, Amy, and Peta—about the differences between healthy and unhealthy, the girls started talking about Natia as someone who was unhealthy because she often brought 'junk' food to school. In another conversation with the same three girls, when asked what an unhealthy lunch looks like, Amy swiftly replied: "Natia's lunch!" These students and another group of girls also complained that Natia often tried to 'scab' food from them (scab is a colloquial term used by the children to describe when someone asks for food or drink). Natia herself told Darren she sometimes 'scabbed' food when she was hungry, a result of either eating her own lunch before school started, giving her lunch to her brother, or having no food for lunch or breakfast in the first place. Natia's perceived inclination to bring chips to school and her tendency to ask other students to share their lunch, combined with her fat body, meant that Natia was understood by others as not only unhealthy, but also immoral—greedy, lazy, a poor chooser, and an irresponsible person.

However, it was clear that Natia and her family struggled with poverty. Natia lived with her mother, father, and four siblings. The family had been living in a three-bedroom 'state house' (one provided and funded by the government through the welfare system), but had recently been evicted and were living in a car at the rear of her cousin's house. There were times when there was no food for her to eat, never mind make a packed lunch and bring it to school (as suggested by the school receptionist). Sometimes Natia was able to get some money from her parents or her auntie and she would buy potato chips (and occasionally a fizzy drink) from her local shop on the way to school—the supermarket was too far away to walk.

She frequently felt guilty about not being able to provide for her brother, embarrassed to ask classmates for food, and shame at not having a healthy lunch like some of her classmates.

## THE GOVERNMENT OF LUNCHES, BODIES, AND BLAME

It is clear that school lunches are shaped by a messy mix of political, social, economic, environmental, historical, and cultural forces. More so, the coupling of lunches with notions of health, fatness, and choice is inextricably interconnected with the ideology of healthism (see Crawford 1980) which shifts the responsibility for health (including body size) onto the individual. By replacing the responsibility for managing (un)healthy behaviors as lying 'within the realm of individual choice' healthism works to foster:

> A continued de-politicization and therefore undermining of the social effort to improve health and well-being … healthism functions as dominant ideology, contributing to the protection of the social order from the examination, critique, and restructuring which would threaten those who benefit from the malaise, misery, and death of others. (Crawford 1980, pp. 368–369)

The notion of healthism reinforces the assumption that children and their families not only *could* take responsibility for their own lunch "choices," but *should* (see Gard 2011). When individuals are *obliged* to take responsibility for their health, they are then able to be *blamed* for making the wrong choices, being irresponsible, and contributing to the 'obesity epidemic'. At the same time, the significant and complex socioeconomic forces that shape food choices, bodies, and health are ignored (see Leahy et al. 2015).

The deliberate endeavor to shape 'the conduct of conduct' of children and parents to specific ends is highly moral. Those who try to govern presume that there 'exists' some type of ideal or normal body, behavior, and/ or thoughts which one should strive to achieve, such as the responsible parent who provides a lunch box filled with nutritious food, the 'good' child who 'chooses' the 'right' food, and those who display a non-fat body. Furthermore, these same governmental actors and institutions also presume that it is possible to structure things so that individuals will do as they are "supposed" to (Scott 1995; Evans 2010). According to Rose (2000, p. 323), government is dependent upon the "unease generated by a normative judgment of what we are and could become" (and what we 'should' become). The moral panic over the threat of obesity has spawned a number of policies, practices, and players in schools (see Gard and Pluim 2014) that attempt to regulate, normalize, and shape certain 'healthy' behaviors (e.g. eating fruit and avoiding junk food), thoughts (e.g. decision-making and willpower), and bodies (especially non-obese bodies). The morality of modern government is further established when individuals understand themselves as being responsible for their own conduct, self-surveillance, self-care, self-regulation, and self-problematization (Dean 2010). In the case of lunch boxes in the United States, New Zealand, and Australia, those who are unable to bring or buy the 'right' type of lunch, or any food at all, are blamed, shamed, and demonized. They are positioned as being "unhealthy on purpose" (Crawford 1984, p. 71).

## CONCLUSION

In this chapter we explore the school lunch box and examine the ways in which it has become a transnational site of surveillance, intervention, and reform. Drawing on the concept of pedagogicalization and a Foucauldian analytical frame, we describe how school lunches act as a kind of normalizing and regulating device to educate on what it means to have an acceptable lunch, behave/consume responsibly, and most importantly embody health. Our analysis reveals the widespread use of the school lunch experience as a (global) strategy to instill ideological and normative messages around health, consumption, and responsibility. Together these messages invoke particular regimes of truth regarding appropriate foods and consumption habits, ideal body forms and functions as well as the schools' justifiable level of intervention to influence these. In many ways the global story of school lunching is not about a few schools in Texas, Lunchbox Blitzing in Australia, young Natia in New Zealand, or the action or intentions of school personnel and policy makers who implement these initiatives—however altruistic they may be. Rather our narrative concerns the ways in which particular rationalities, ideologies, and discourses (occurring in multiple sites) can be levied to form and constitute particular modes of being and justify potentially programmatic and/or harmful action.

## NOTE

1. In New Zealand, Pākehā is a common Māori word to describe immigrants to New Zealand of European descent.

# REFERENCES

Bell, A., & Swinburn, B. (2004). What are the key food groups to target for preventing obesity and improving nutrition in schools? *European Journal of Clinical Nutrition, 58*, 258–263.

Bernstein, B. (2001). From pedagogies to knowledges. In A. M. Morais, B. Davies, & H. Daniels (Eds.), *Towards a sociology of pedagogy: The contribution of Basil Bernstein to research* (pp. 363–368). New York: Peter Lang.

Burrow, A. (2015, March 24). *Kids' lunch should come from parents.* Retrieved from http://www.stuff.co.nz

Burrows, L., & Wright, J. (2007). Prescribing practices: Shaping healthy children in schools. *International Journal of Children's Rights, 15*(1), 1–16.

Castel, R. (1991). From dangerousness to risk. In G. Burchell, C. Gordon, & P. Miller (Eds.), *The Foucault effect: Studies in governmentality* (pp. 281–289). Chicago: University of Chicago Press.

Chorley, M. (2015, July 1). *Daily mail.* Retrieved from http://www.dailymail. co.uk/news/article-3145629/Teachers-confiscate-unhealthy-food-Government-issues-rules-carry-lunchbox-inspections.html

Counihan, C., & Van Esterik, P. (2012). *Food and culture: A reader.* New York: Routledge.

Crawford, R. (1980). Healthism and the medicalization of everyday life. *International Journal of Health Services, 10*, 365–388.

Crawford, R. (1984). A cultural account of "health": Control, release, and the social body. In J. McKinley (Ed.), *Issues in the political economy of health care* (pp. 66–103). London: Tavistock.

Dean, M. (2002). Powers of life and death beyond governmentality. *Cultural Values, 6*(1–2), 119–138.

Dean, M. (2010). *Governmentality: Power and rule in modern society* (2nd ed.). London: Sage.

Department of Education and Early Childhood Development. (2012). *Healthy Canteen Kit: School canteens and other school food services policy.* Melbourne: State Government Victoria.

Dolby, N., & Rizvi, F. (Eds.). (2008). *Youth moves: Identities and education in global perspectives.* New York: Routledge.

Eng, M., & Hood. J. (2011, April 11). Chicago bans some lunches brought from home. *Chicago Tribune.* Retrieved from http://articles.chicagotribune. com/2011-04-11/news/ct-met-school-lunch-restrictions-041120110410_1_lunch-food-provider-public-school

Evans, B. (2010). Anticipating fatness: Childhood, affect and the pre-emptive 'war on obesity'. *Transactions of the Institute of British Geographers, 35*(1), 21–38.

Flowers, R., & Swan, E. (2011). 'Eating at us': Representations of knowledge in the activist documentary film Food, Inc. *Studies in the Education of Adults, 43*(2), 234–250.

Flowers, R., & Swan, E. (2012). Pedagogies of doing good: Problematisations, authorities, technologies and teleologies in food activism. *Australian Journal of Adult Learning, 52*, 532–572.

Flowers, R., & Swan, E. (2015). Food pedagogies: Histories, definitions and moralities. In R. Flowers & E. Swan (Eds.), *Food pedagogies* (pp. 1–27). Farnham: Ashgate.

Forsyth, J. (2011, May 13). Cameras in Texas schools to keep eyes on fries. *Reuters*. Retrieved from http://www.reuters.com/article/us-food-cafeterias-cameras-odd-idUSTRE74C3AH20110513?feedType=RSS&feedName=oddly EnoughNews&utm_source=feedburner&utm_medium=feed&utm_campaign =Feed%3A+reuters%2FoddlyEnoughNews+%28News+%2F+US+%2F+Oddly+ Enough%29

Foucault, M. (2003). The subject and power. In P. Rabinow & N. S. Rose (Eds.), *The essential Foucault: Selections from essential works of Foucault, 1954–1984* (pp. 126–144). New York: New Press.

Gard, M. (2011). *The end of the obesity epidemic*. Oxon: Routledge.

Gard, M., & Pluim, C. (2014). *Schools and public health: Past, present and future*. Lanham: Lexington Books.

Gibson, K., & Dempsey, S. (2015). Make good choices, kid: Biopolitics of children's bodies and school lunch reform in Jamie Oliver's Food Revolution. *Children's Geographies, 13*, 44–58.

Harman, V., & Cappellini, B. (2017). Lunchboxes, health, leisure and well-being: Analysing the connections. In Z. Benkő, I. Modi, & K. Tarkó (Eds.), *Leisure, health and well-being: A holistic approach* (pp. 45–60). Basingstoke: Palgrave Macmillan.

Kelly, P. (2000). The dangerousness of youth-at-risk: The possibilities of surveillance and intervention in uncertain times. *Journal of Adolescence, 23*(4), 463–476.

Lawlis, T., Knox, M., & Jamieson, M. (2016). School canteens: A systematic review of the policy, perceptions and use from an Australian perspective. *Nutrition and Dietetics, 73*(4), 389–398.

Leahy, D. (2009). Disgusting pedagogies. In J. Wright & V. Hardwick (Eds.), *Biopolitics and the 'obesity epidemic': Governing bodies* (pp. 172–182). New York: Routledge.

Leahy, D. (2014). Assembling a health [y] subject: Risky and shameful pedagogies in health education. *Critical Public Health, 24*, 171–181.

Leahy, D., Gray, E., Cutter-Mackenzie, A., & Eames, C. (2015). Schooling food in contemporary times: Taking stock. *Australian Journal of Environmental Education, 31*, 1–11.

Levine, S. (2010). *School lunch politics: The surprising history of America's favorite welfare program*. New York: Princeton University Press.

Li, T. M. (2007). *The will to improve: Governmentality, development, and the practice of politics*. Durham: Duke University Press.

74    C. PLUIM ET AL.

Lunchbox Blitz. (n.d.). Retrieved from http://www.lunchboxblitz.com/. Accessed 6 Mar 2017.

Mackey-Kallis, S., & Hahn, D. F. (1991). Questions of public will and private action: The power of the negative in the Reagans "Just Say No" morality campaign. *Communication Quarterly, 39*(1), 1–17.

Miller, P., & Rose, N. (2008). *Governing the present.* Cambridge, UK: Polity.

Nukaga, M. (2008). The underlife of kids' school lunchtime negotiating ethnic boundaries and identity in food exchange. *Journal of Contemporary Ethnography, 37*(3), 342–380.

Osborne, T. (1997). Of health and statecraft. In A. Petersen & R. Bunton (Eds.), *Foucault, health and medicine* (pp. 173–188). New York: Routledge.

Peters, M., & Marshall, J. (1996). *Individualism and community: Education and social policy in the postmodern condition.* London: Falmer Press.

Petersen, A. (1997). Risk, governance and the new public health. In A. Petersen & R. Bunton (Eds.), *Foucault, health and medicine* (pp. 189–206). New York: Routledge.

Pike, J., & Leahy, D. (2012). School food and the pedagogies of parenting. *Australian Journal of Adult Learning, 52*(3), 434–459.

Powell, D. (2015). *'Part of the solution'?: Charities, corporate philanthropy and healthy lifestyles education in New Zealand primary schools.* Unpublished doctoral dissertation. Charles Sturt University, Bathurst.

Rich, E., & Evans, J. (2005). 'Fat ethics' – The obesity discourse and body politics. *Social Theory and Health, 3*(4), 341–358.

Rose, N. (2000). Government and control. *British Journal of Criminology, 40*, 321–339.

Rosenbaum, D. P., & Hanson, G. S. (1998). Assessing the effects of school-based drug education: A six-year multilevel analysis of project DARE. *Journal of Research in Crime and Delinquency, 35*(4), 381–412.

Sanigorski, A., Bell, A., Kremer, P., & Swinburn, B. (2005). Lunchbox contents of Australian school children: Room for improvement. *European Journal of Clinical Nutrition, 59*, 1310–1316.

Schee, V. (2004). The privatization of food services in schools: Undermining children's health, social equity, and democratic education. In D. Boyles (Ed.), *Schools or markets? Commercialism, privatization, and school business partnerships* (pp. 1–30). New York: Lawrence Erlbaum.

Scott, D. (1995). Colonial governmentality. *Social Text, 43*, 191–220.

Welch, R., McMahon, S., & Wright, J. (2012). The medicalisation of food pedagogies in primary schools and popular culture: A case for awakening subjugated knowledges. *Discourse: Studies in the Cultural Politics of Education, 33*(5), 713–728.

# CHAPTER 5

# "Eating Democracy": School Lunch and the Social Meaning of Eating in Critical Times

*Paula M. Salvio*

## INTRODUCTION

Early in December 1940, the United States National Research Council, in collaboration with anthropologist Ruth Benedict, and at the request of the National Defense Advisory Commission, established the Committee on Food Habits. Benedict was enlisted because she had a special interest in the cultural aspects of nutrition and brought to the committee her knowledge of the links between culture and personality. She also had her own motive, which was to garner for anthropology some of the prestige of "science" associated with the Research Council. The National Defense Advisory Commission had requested the formation of a committee to study the physical health and nutrition of the US population, because they increasingly viewed malnutrition, exacerbated during the Depression and existing among large segments of the population, as a threat to national security. Improving nutrition was fast becoming a major federal concern. The express intentions of the Committee on Food Habits were to assess the social implications of wartime adjustment to food conditions, to promote nutrition among a range of social groups, and to establish long-term nutritious eating habits.

P. M. Salvio (✉)
University of New Hampshire, Durham, NH, USA

© The Author(s) 2018
S. Rice, A. G. Rud (eds.), *Educational Dimensions of School Lunch*,
https://doi.org/10.1007/978-3-319-72517-8_5

Margaret Mead joined Benedict in January 1942, having previously worked closely with Benedict and Franz Boas, both of whom were identified with the anthropological school of thought referred to as "culture and personality." Through Benedict's intervention, Mead became Executive Director of the Committee and directed the office in Washington, DC until 1945. Combining her interests in institutional food with a specific focus on school lunch programs, Mead began to establish an applied research agenda for the Committee that sought to reorganize thinking about food. The school lunch menu, argued Mead, should "transform diverse ethnic food cultures into a national identity" (Levine 2008, p. 68), "particularly in times of crisis" (p. 66). While Mead insisted that "[e]very child eating in school and every adult eating in a public cafeteria ... should be comfortable with the food offerings," she also insisted that cafeteria planners ensure a nutritious menu, which might mean offering foods different from those eaten at home (Levine 2008, p. 68). How to balance nutrition, sensitivity to ethnic or religious diversity, and resources allocated to feeding the public was the question. Mead decided that a bland homogeneity would be better than an expensive and potentially divisive heterogeneity. "Because of the great diversity of food differences in the United States," Mead observed, "it is more practicable to try to establish feeding patterns which do not offend any group." School lunchrooms and other cafeterias, she suggested, should offer only "food that is fairly innocuous and has low emotional value" (Levine 2008, p. 68). Menus should be planned with as little "distinctive flavoring as possible" (Levine 2008, p. 68). In fact, "the only seasoning Mead recommended was salt. All others she said, would alienate one group or another" (Levine 2008, p. 68).

Mead's views and the work of the Committee raise several questions. What are the ethical and pedagogical implications of serving food with "low emotional value"? What does it mean to build a national identity through food pathways that diminish the variety and intensity of gustatory experiences? This chapter opens the archive of the US school lunch in an effort to more fully explore the relationships among eating, emotional life, and democracy, and how these relationships informed and continue to inform US public school lunch programs.

My reading of the Committee on Food Habits, led by Mead, is informed by D.W. Winnicott's concepts of potential space and transitional objects, and Hannah Arendt's concept of "enlarged mentality" (1968b). For Winnicott (1964), the eater is not a fully constituted subject, but is continually in the process of being constituted through their orientations toward food. Food always has the potential to reconstitute the subject, gradually introducing a taste for the social world outside the self. I argue that Mead's approach to cultivating a national identity through the school lunch program paradoxically diminished the potential that food and mealtime had for inviting students to experience more capacious, social, and transcultural worlds. I suggest that her approach narrowed rather than broadened the boundaries of cultural selves and that it foreclosed on the potential food has for refining the diverse sensual perceptions and tastes that are vital to an education committed to cultivating the "enlarged mentality" Arendt so highly valued. For Arendt, the capacity to represent others' perspectives through the faculty of imagination was necessary for educating a politically engaged democratic citizenry.

## "EATING IN AMERICA IS PRIMARILY A SUPER-EGO PROBLEM"

On December 11, 1942, Margaret Mead spoke to the Topeka Psychoanalytic Society about the research findings of the Committee on Food Habits. Having recently accepted the position of Executive Director of the Committee, she hoped that by outlining several of the findings, psychoanalysts might find it worthwhile to collaborate with the Committee in conducting research in the formation of food habits (Mead 1942, 1943a). Drawing on interview data with the public, reports from nutrition experts, studies of the symbolism used in advertising, and random qualitative opinion sampling, Mead reported on the findings that "eating in America is primarily a 'super-ego' problem," that is tied up with questions of morality. Mead (1943a) described this problem in the following way:

> if you eat enough of the food that is not good but is good for you, you are then permitted to eat a little of the food that is good but is not good for you. This attitude is instilled into each generation by the use of reward and punishment and as a result the findings of the science of nutrition do not become an automatic part of our cultural tradition but remain a subject of moral choice for each individual. (pp. 45–46)

According to Mead, the studies showed how cultural attitudes sustained a tension between the ideal of nutritious food and the desire for gustatory pleasure. The Committee concluded that in the average American household, food was the site of conflict, coercion, and, surprisingly, the assertion of masculinity. Despite her personal unconventionality, as a public spokesperson, Mead analyzed this site along conventional gender lines. Given that men and children tend not to like vegetables, she explained, women find themselves in the position of having to trick and cajole them. Desserts are used as bribes. Raiding the fridge and eating too many sweets are experienced as small victories over food taboos set by the mother and wife. Violating such taboos, argued Mead (1942), allowed men and children to exercise a form of independence from the "feminine" and offered delight in a naughty pleasure rather than a feeling of guilty conscience. Setting the scene of eating habits in psychoanalytic terms, Mead concluded that appealing to one's conscience in order to establish healthy eating habits might be necessary, but certainly not sufficient. How, Mead asked, is the unconscious involved in forming food habits in the American character structure?

That food and eating are experienced as moral issues—good food versus bad food or healthy food versus tasty food—also worked to undermine the capacity to experience eating as a sensual pleasure. In their interviews with men, women, and children throughout the country, Mead and her colleagues found that descriptions of eating as a sensual experience were absent. When asked about favorite foods, the Committee found that people would respond with overgeneralized words, such as steak or ice cream, and emphasized the appearance of food rather than how it tasted. Mead (1942) proposed to the psychoanalysts she was addressing in Topeka that they study the developmental process of eating, and when it became delibidinized and established as a "super-ego problem." In other words, Mead recommended studies that explored when people ceased to take pleasure in eating.

At the end of her talk, Mead (1942) asked her audience at the Psychoanalytic Society to expand the project of psychodynamics to include studies of groups of people at a specific epoch in history so that their ideas could be made "available for social planning." "It would be tragic," argued Mead,

> if this wealth of insight were not to be made so available. The successful application of psychoanalytic theory and techniques to the solution of any one present day problem – such as that of altering American food habits to preserve nutritional standards in the midst of war shortages – would pave the way for a more widespread contribution to the pressing social problems of the times. (p. 50)

Among the most pressing problems facing Mead and her colleagues was how to make unappealing, uncommon, unfamiliar, protein-rich foods appealing to a nutritionally deprived population, given that most of the domestic meat was being shipped overseas to feed soldiers and allies (Wansink 2002).

Working closely with the social psychologist Kurt Lewin, whose expertise was in the area of groups and group dynamics, Mead came to believe that in order to change food habits, an understanding of what prevented people from eating certain foods (disincentives) as well as educating the gatekeeping cook about food preparation was necessary. Additionally, the process of learning to assimilate unfamiliar foods into a daily diet had to be grounded in an understanding of nutrition science. In his study of the Committee on Food Habits, Brian Wansink (2002) found that the research sponsored by the Committee on Food Habits organized acceptable food around four themes: "a food must be 1) selected, 2) available, 3) familiar and 4) exactly as expected (i.e. safe)" (pp. 91–92). Mead directed several studies that examined food selection in school cafeterias throughout the country. She came to believe that the school lunchroom could become a place to promote democracy as well as be a model for eating that mirrored middle-class values, what she described as a "well-regulated family group" (Levine 2008, p. 67). Under Mead's leadership, each small round table in the school cafeteria was assigned a "host" and "hostess" who led the meal according to the social norms privileged in the Anglo-American household. Quiet environments were encouraged, as well as "table courtesies," that included lessons in etiquette, nutrition, and conversation (Levine 2008, p. 67).

Striking about Mead's understanding of food and culture are the contradictions that surface between her lecture to the Topeka Psychoanalytic Society and her public representation of the research conducted with the Committee on Food Habits and recommendations for school lunch programs. During her talk in Topeka, she recognized the role the unconscious plays with respect to taste and eating, and how important the libidinal pleasures associated with seeing, hearing, tasting, smelling, and touching food are in determining what one eats (Mead 1942). Yet her approach to cultivating democracy in the lunchroom limited a range of tastes and abided by a scientific approach to eating and nutrition associated with the mental hygiene movement that failed to capture the diverse appetites of the populations living in the United States.

In a 1946 edition of *Hygeia: The Health Magazine of the American Medical Association*, Mead is quoted by Thomas C. Desmond as promoting a balanced diet. "In reorganizing our habits of thinking about food," Desmond wrote when paraphrasing Mead, "we must not develop the habit of eating more spinach, but a habit of mind which demands a balanced meal... Our daily diet should be as nourishing and balanced as the existing science of nutrition can make it" (p. 202). Inherent in the message Mead delivered about nutrition during the war was a call for a strong, highly developed super-ego that made rational, scientifically informed decisions about what to eat. Again, this call, which clearly represents Mead's and her colleagues' intentions to cure and to emancipate the US population from poor nutrition, is in direct contradiction to her talk in Topeka, where she underscores that eating in the United States is a "superego problem." I want to take a moment to reflect on her claim when speaking to the psychoanalytic society given that the aim of the Committee on Food Habits was to cure the US population of poor health and to emancipate them, as I stated earlier, from what was understood as poor eating habits.

In *Disavowed Knowledge: Psychoanalysis, Education, and Teaching*, Peter M. Taubman (2012) argues that both education and psychoanalysis are characterized by a split between a therapeutic project, which he describes as the desire to cure coupled with aspirations for scientific certainty, and an emancipatory project, which he describes as the desire to deepen and to understand our inner lives, without the certainty that our lives will indeed be more fulfilling or happy. Following Taubman, I would like to suggest that under Mead's leadership, the school lunch program can be read as part of a larger history of education's disavowal of the emancipatory project and its association with the mental hygiene movement, a point I address in the following section of this chapter. While Mead was deeply involved with psychoanalysis in her role as an anthropologist, particularly in her work with the Menninger Clinic, her work on the Committee on Food Habits suggests she shared the very ambivalence experienced by so many educators about using psychoanalysis to educate the public and to pursue insights into what constitutes a meaningful life. This disavowal was tied to an ambivalence about recognizing the unconscious as a vital, generative part of our psychic lives. It is important to note that despite their attempts to approach their charge with scientific precision, the Committee on Food Habits was never quite successful.

In her study of the history of the school lunch program, Levine (2008) points out that given the extent to which nutritionists and home economists worked to appeal to the national public to eat better, it is unlikely that balanced meals actually appeared on many American dinner plates (p. 65). In other words, changing food habits was not a clear-cut, conscious project. Nor was the day-to-day practice of eating balanced meals affordable or practical. Levine cites food writer M.F.K. Fisher as criticizing the idea of "balanced meals," and describing the National Recommended Daily Allotment (RDA) charts and recommendations as "one of the stupidest things in an earnest but stupid school of culinary thought." Fisher was even more critical of the idea of creating monthly menu plans, arguing that it was difficult enough to prepare even one tasty meal a day, given the labor and the cost (p. 66). Nonetheless, the principles of the RDA were the guiding force behind the national school lunch program and they continued to guide the work of Mead and her colleagues.

Combined with the principles of the RDA were the principles of a democratic practice that included a respect for personal choice (Levine 2008). For this reason, the Committee on Food Habits worked to play down the differences that characterized ethnic Americans in order to create a unified national identity. The Committee recommended that school lunch include "low toned foods" such as plain soups, chicken, plain rice, boiled spaghetti, and potatoes (p. 68). In addition to food that had "low emotional value," Mead and her colleagues recommended that the most essential feature of the school lunch should be choice. Mead argued that the ability to have and to make choices was a sign of being an adult in a democracy, and to reduce choice would be to relegate the adult to the status of a child (p. 68).

The sounds of Mead's call for choice in the lunchroom can still be heard today, although in a neoliberal era. The right to choose high-sugar sweets and heavily salted fries and chips has been rhetorically recast by anti-government figures such as Sarah Palin and Glen Beck. According to Palin and Beck, the right to choose fast food and foods high in glucose and salt is integral to the American way of life, the pursuit of happiness, and the integrity of the family. Figures such as Beck and Palin know how to appeal to the appetites of their audience. In 2010, *The New York Times* reported that Palin appeared at an elementary school in Pennsylvania with platters of cookies to argue that the Obama "nanny state" is "essentially, snatching cookies – i.e., the pursuit of happiness- from the mouths of babes"

(Warner 2010). Beck has a litany of complaints against government involvement in nutrition. In the same *New York Times* report, Beck is described as criticizing the "choice architects" of the Obama administration for believing "you're incapable of making decisions...left to your own devices, you're going to eat too much, you're going to be a big fat fatty." Indeed, notes Warner, the author of the *Times* report, the cookies are pushing back among the anti-government insurgent, "like the return of the repressed."

Almost 80 years after Mead began her work on the Committee on Food Habits, the challenge of waging war on poor nutritional habits in the United States continues. While Mead's challenge was poverty, war, and malnutrition, and the contemporary challenge today is tied to agribusiness and corporate involvement in the production of fast food, both efforts faced the challenge of how to change eating behaviors in the context of a complex and diverse set of food cultures, politics, and emotional lives. The US population continues to suffer with health problems, although today threats to health are tied to a different form of malnutrition—obesity. (More than two-thirds of American adults are obese or overweight, and 17 percent of children and adolescents are obese. Obesity will become the single most preventable cause of premature death in the United States, a condition historically linked to smoking [Hurt et al. 2010].) School lunch programs throughout the United States are hardly uniform, but they continue to be inflected with many of the features promoted by Mead, including the importance of choice and attention to nutrition. What is ironically absent given Mead's work as an anthropologist closely associated with psychoanalysis is the lack of psychoanalytic research to study, as she so eloquently pointed out to her audience in Topeka, the libidinal qualities of food and eating and how to break old cycles of association—warm bread with a safe home—with new associations that combine nutritious food with respect for diverse appetites and tastes.

I will now turn to the scholarship of Winnicott and Arendt in an effort to more fully ground the limitations of Mead's approach to the social meaning of eating in critical times. I argue that her limitations are grounded in her failure to recognize the generative role the unconscious might play in understanding food habits as well as in her alliance with the mental hygiene movement. In my estimation, the limited achievements of the school lunch program under Mead's leadership are tied to her feelings of ambivalence about the emancipatory and therapeutic projects in education and psychoanalysis, and this ambivalence plays out in her approaches to educate the public about nutrition and eating. Today, the majority of students in the United States attending public schools, particularly schools in underserved neighborhoods, have inherited not only a school lunch legacy that lacks nutrition and flavor, but also a school lunch program that lacks a relationship with local communities that might serve as vibrant sources of nourishment and gustatory pleasure.

## EATING IN THE NAME OF "SOCIAL ADJUSTMENT"

In his 1936 essay "Appetite and Emotional Disorder," Winnicott noted that "the study of psychology has been obscured by our lack of control over physical disease, and by our ignorance about diet" (p. 417). Drawing on years of careful history-taking of his patients, Winnicott explores the role that food plays in understanding the psychosocial subject, and proposes that children often use their doubt about food to disguise their doubt about love. And doubt about food, as Adam Phillips (2009) notes in a reading of Winnicott's position, correlates to doubt about resources and fears of deprivation. In *Making Sense of Taste: Food and Philosophy*, Carolyn Korsmeyer (1999) also emphasizes that because tasting and eating alter one's very constitution,

> their exercise requires trust. We must trust that our foods are healthful and not poison, and thus we rely not only on the quality of the objects to be eaten but also on the kindly disposition of our eating companions and those who are responsible for preparing our food. (p. 189)

Rejecting food, finding it abject or disgusting, is often the key negative effect, not only for the child refusing to eat, but for anyone rejecting the food culture of others. According to Winnicott, food is the first "not-me" object experienced by the baby, and it is through small doses of food that the baby begins to experience all that is new, foreign, and unfamiliar and develops a taste for the social world beyond the self (Winnicott 1958; Salvio 2012). Given Winnicott's findings, what are the implications of preparing school lunches that not only contain a "low emotional value," but reject the tastes, local affiliations, smells, and appetites of the diverse populations of students attending public school during the war (Salvio 2012, 2016)?

Mead's culinary practices in the lunchroom, read as part of the mental hygiene movement (which was a branch of the progressive education movement), worked to deliberately educate the super-ego vis-à-vis scientific approaches to nutrition and education that promoted "normality," health, and cure, and inadvertently contributed to the "medicalization" of American education (Taubman 2012). Combining psychoanalysis, the child-centered strand of progressive education, with John Dewey's scientific methods of inquiry, the mental hygienists hoped to build a more democratic society and a healthier person. Following the tenets of mental hygienists, Mead's lunchroom curriculum promoted "social adjustment" by privileging the structure of the nuclear family, and heterosexual relationships, as made evident in the practices of etiquette and hosting called for at Mead's lunchroom table. And while the mental hygiene movement was informed by psychoanalysis, the psychoanalytic traditions that influenced them valued a medical model that promoted individual health in the service of social cohesion and secure personhood, and understood the unconscious as a cesspool that should be adjusted rather than a radical force that subverts the belief in certainty, mastery, or complete control. In fact, Mead promoted the idea of food with "low emotional value" to secure social cohesion. In 1948, three years after she had joined the US National Committee for Mental Hygiene, Mead delivered a paper titled "Collective Guilt" wherein she argued that the family mediated between the individual and culture (1948b). Following her work with Benedict, Mead (1948a) was tireless in showing—both in her research and through her work in public policy—how the personality traits characteristic of a nation could be attributed to the family socialization in various cultures. Like her colleagues active in the progressive educational project, Mead believed in a liberal path to progress. On the personal level, this could be attained by achieving what she described as normal relationships and a capacity for self-expression. On the social level, progress was attained through social adaptation, a sense of responsibility, and equal relations among individuals. Mental hygienists such as Mead had great faith that through direct interventions in behavior that created "healthy personalities and character structures," a healthy social order could be established and sustained (Frank 1948a,b, p. 58).

Yet, her belief in the unconscious was absent from any official project she executed as Director of the Committee on Food Habits. As well, the approaches she took to feeding students in school and to nutrition education actually contributed to the "super-ego" problem she presented to the Topeka Psychoanalytic Institute. The school lunch legacy we have inherited today carries with it the very anxieties that Winnicott outlined in 1936. The doubt students and teachers have about the food served in the school cafeteria can be read as an expression of the profound lack of love, pleasure, and resources offered through institutional projects such as the school lunch.

If Mead was initially correct that the challenge of educating the US population about nutrition was a "super-ego problem" tied, in part, to practices of preparing food and eating that were devoid of libidinal energy, then what might it mean to take up Mead's initial challenge posed to the Topeka Psychoanalytic Institute and study when food is delibidinized and what libidinizing food preparation and eating might look like?

Taubman (2012) argued that as psychoanalytic theory became less speculative and lost its grounding in the humanities, it paradoxically lost its libido, a claim that applies directly to Mead's approach to establishing the school lunch program. By aligning the school lunch program with a mental hygiene curriculum that privileged a scientific approach to preparing and eating food, the psychic energy that animates life and demands pleasure was denied a place at Mead's lunchroom table. Moreover, by promoting food with "low emotional value," food that was devoid of distinctive tastes, Mead's approach to the school lunch failed to cultivate the ability of student-citizens to take on the perspectives of others as well as the sensitivity required to determine what might be in the interest of all members of a democratic polity. For Arendt, judgments must combine principled commitment with a keen sensitivity to the specific circumstances in which they are made. The emphasis Arendt (1958) placed on appreciating diverse perspectives is expressed below:

> Being seen and being heard by others derive their significance from the fact that everybody sees and hears from a different position. This is the meaning of public life. ... Only where things can be seen by many in a variety of aspects without changing their identity, so that those who are gathered around them know they see sameness in utter diversity, can worldly reality truly and reliably appear... The end of the common world has come when it is seen only under one aspect and is permitted to present itself in only one perspective. (pp. 57–58)

Inherent in Mead's commitment to using the school lunch to create a national identity was the unintended consequence of undermining rather than cultivating an appreciation for diverse perspectives that would lead, not to the preservation of individuals' beliefs in what is good for them as individuals, but to a shift in perspectives that had the capacity to lead to pursuing a substantive good that would sustain plurality. Such a project cannot be reduced to a formula or be easily measured. Rather, Arendt believed that a person with an "enlarged mentality" can shift her ground in order to appreciate the standpoint of others. In other words, Arendt asked that we think beyond a politics of self-interest. "To think with an enlarged mentality," writes Arendt (1982), "means that one trains one's imagination to go visiting" (p. 43). An enlarged mentality connects closely with the specificity of a situation with particular conditions of the standpoints that one must understand in order to arrive at a "general standpoint" (p. 44). This capacity might also be understood as a form of thinking that brings together aesthetics—an ability to imagine the positions of others who are absent—with the exercise of critical judgment that takes into account a diverse set of standpoints, rather than aiming, as I noted earlier, for a universal standpoint for all. Arendt (1968a) explains the way in which political thought is representational in the following passage:

> I form an opinion by considering a given issue from different viewpoints, by making present to my mind the standpoints of those who are absent; that is, I represent them. This process of representation does not blindly adopt the actual views of those who stand somewhere else, and hence look upon the world from a different perspective; that is a question neither of empathy, as though I tried to be or feel like somebody else, nor of counting noses and joining a majority but of being and thinking in my own identity where actually I am not. The more people's standpoints I have present in my mind while I am pondering a given issue, the better I can imagine how I would feel and think in their place, the stronger will be my capacity for representative thinking and the more valued my final conclusions, my opinion. (p. 241)

Rather than promoting generalized thinking or a generalized conception of citizenship that is wedded to a universal model of justice for all, Arendt called for a plurality of voices to be recognized. Considering the perspectives of others at the lunchroom table might begin with opportunities to appreciate the social embeddedness and historical conditions that influence food preparation and the social experiences of eating together in critical times.

What might a school lunch curriculum look like that engages in an emancipatory project tied to the humanities? In my estimation, a public school lunch that includes a wide range of tastes and engages communities in accessing and preparing food holds the promise of promoting a form of citizenship that cares about particularized others—their traditions, pleasures, and appetites—rather than a liberal project that promotes self-interest and an abstract unified national identity that excludes those whose needs and interests are not likely to be heard. "Eating together," writes Carolyn Korsmeyer (1999),

> is a common signal among most peoples for friendship, truce, or celebration... but just how common eating transforms itself from fuel to feast, from satisfaction of need to social bond, may not always be obvious...What I have summarized as the intimacy of eating is part of what knits together those who eat – the mutual trust presumed, the social equality of those who sit down together, and the shared tastes and pleasures of the table. Shared eating is commonly recognized as among the most enjoyable aspects of civilized food preparation and consumption, but what in fact must be presumed, subdued, or accomplished for this "civilized" activity to be possible? (pp. 187–188)

Susan Laird has written eloquently about the pedagogical implications of Korsmeyer's philosophical study of literary narratives of eating. Turning to several archives of school lunch narratives, including *The Dewey School* (1936), Louisa May Alcott's fictional school Plumfield (1868–1870), and Alice Waters' Edible Schoolyards Project, Laird (2013) challenges educators to consider school lunch as a "curriculum laboratory worthy of imaginative efforts to rethink and reconstruct" (p. 14). In closing, I would like to suggest that the teacher education curriculum take the school lunch seriously, rather than treating it as a trivial event. Both Korsmeyer (1999) and Laird (2013) remind us that philosophy/philosophy of education has long neglected taste and the enjoyments of eating. Reflection on taste and rituals of cooking and eating together hold the promise of leading to democratic practices that cultivate an appreciation and respect for the standpoints of others as well as to the unique singularity that is constituted by a radically other unconscious. In opening ourselves up to the unconscious, we might work toward exploring the enigmas of our existence and the ways in which our hungers, appetites, tastes, and desire for nourishment shape what it means to prepare food and to eat together in critical times.

REFERENCES

Arendt, H. (1958). *The human condition.* Chicago: University of Chicago Press.

Arendt, H. (1965). *Basic moral propositions.* University of Chicago Hannah Arendt Papers, Library of Congress, Container 40, p. 024648.

Arendt, H. (1968a). *Between past and future: Eight exercises in political thought.* New York: Penguin Books.

Arendt, H. (1968b). *Totalitarianism: Part III of the origins of totalitarianism.* New York: Harcourt, Inc..

Arendt, H. (1982). In R. Beiner (Ed.), *Lectures on Kant's political philosophy.* Chicago: University of Chicago Press.

Desmond, T. C. (1946). In your meals. *Hygeia: The Journal of Health of the American Medical Association, 24*(1–6), 200–202.

Flammang, J. A. (2009). *A taste for civilization: Food, politics and civil society.* Chicago: University of Illinois Press.

Frank, L. K. (1948a). *Projective methods.* Springfield, IL: C.C. Thomas.

Frank, L. K. (1948b). *Society as the patient: Essays on culture and personality.* New York, NY: Verso.

Hurt, R. T., Kulisek, C., Buchanan, L., & McClave, S. (2010). The obesity epidemic: Challenges, health initiatives, and implications for gastroenterologists. *Gastroenterology & Hepatology: The Independent Peer Reviewed Journal, 6*(12), 780–792.

Korsmeyer, C. (1999). *Making sense of taste: Food and philosophy.* Ithaca/London: Cornell University Press.

Korsmeyer, C. (Ed.). (2005). *The taste culture reader: Experiencing food and drink.* London/Oxford: Bloomsbury Publishing.

Laird, S. (2013). Bringing educational thought to public school lunch: Alice Waters and the edible school yard. *Journal of Thought, 48*(2), 12–27.

Levine, S. (2008). *School lunch politics: The surprising history of America's favorite welfare program.* Princeton: Princeton University Press.

Mead, M. (1942). The problem of changing food habits: With suggestions for psychoanalytic contributions. *Bulletin of the Menninger Clinic, 7*(2), 20–31.

Mead, M. (1943a). The problem of changing food habits: With suggestions for psychoanalytic contributions. Reprinted in *Institute of General Semantics, 1* (1), 47–50.

Mead, M. (1943b). Dietary patterns and food habits. *Journal of the American Dietetic Association, 19,* 1–5.

Mead, M. (1943c). The factor of food habits. *The Annals of the American Academy of Political and Social Science, 4,* 21–57.

Mead, M. (1945a). Significant aspects of regional food patterns. Fifth Session: Regional vs. National Food Habits and Nutrition, Committee on Food Habits (mimeograph).

Mead, M. (1945b). Nutritional status and food consumption of rural children in Oregon. Sixth Session: The Relation Between Food Consumption Habits and Nutritional Status, Committee on Food Habits (mimeograph).

Mead, M. (1945c). *Manual for the study of food habits: Report of the committee on food habits. Bulletin of the National Research Council*, No. 111. Washington, DC: National Academy of Sciences.

Mead, M. (1948a). Cultural contexts of nutritional patterns. *Science, 108*(2813), 598–599.

Mead, M. (1948b). *Collective Guilt*. In Proceedings of the International Conference in Medical Psychotherapy, pp. 57–65. The conference was a part of the International Congress on Mental Health, London, 1948, and the volume is the third of the four-volume series International Congress on Mental Health, London, 1948, edited by J.C. Flugel et al.

Phillips, A. (2009). Insatiable creatures. *The Guardian*. Retrieved from https://www.theguardian.com/books/2009/aug/08/excess-adam-phillips

Probyn, E. (2000). *Carnal appetites: Food sex identities*. London/New York: Routledge.

Salvio, P. M. (2012). Dishing it out: Food blogs and post-feminist domesticity. *Gastronomica: The Journal of Food and Culture, 12*(3), 31–39.

Salvio, P. M. (2013). Exercising the 'Right to Research': Youth-based community media production as transformative action. *English in Education, 47*(2), 163–180.

Salvio, P. M. (2016). A taste of justice: Digital media and Libera Terra's antimafia public pedagogy of agrarian dissent. In R. Pickering-Iazzi (Ed.), *The Italian antimafia, new media and the culture of legality* (pp. 85–101). Toronto: University of Toronto Press.

Slayton, R. A. (1986). *Back of the yards: The making of a local democracy*. Chicago: The University of Chicago Press.

Taubman, P. M. (2012). *Disavowed knowledge: Psychoanalysis, education, and teaching*. New York, NY: Routledge.

Wansink, B. (2002). Changing eating habits on the home front: Lost lessons from World War II research. *Journal of Public Policy and Marketing, 21*(1), 90–99.

Warner, J. (2010). Junking Junk Food. *The New York Times*. Retrieved from http://www.nytimes.com/2010/11/28/magazine/28FOB-wwln-t.html

Winnicott, D. W. (1958). Originally published in *Collected papers: Through pediatrics to psycho-analysis* (pp. 33–51). London: Tavistock.

Winnicott, D. W. (1964). *The child, the family and the outside world*. Harmondsworth: Penguin.

Winnicott, D. W. (1974). *Playing and reality*. Harmondsworth: Penguin.

CHAPTER 6

# Food for a Common(s) Curriculum: Learning to Recognize and Resist Food Enclosures

*John J. Lupinacci and Alison Happel-Parkins*

Amid the complicated and often industrial landscapes of education, there exist examples of curriculum and pedagogy that breathe life into the potential of diverse, socially just, and sustainable communities. With our attention on what educators and schools can do to support students experiencing social and environmental injustice, we turn to food. More specifically, in this chapter we focus on what we, as educators and educational researchers, can learn from efforts to resist what we call food enclosures, in Detroit, Michigan. From these efforts we examine the ways in which this movement to recognize and resist food insecurity can spur educators to think about addressing important twenty-first-century challenges—such as food security and food enclosures. The term "food enclosures" refers to Western industrial socio-political and economic arrangements that limit access to the production, preparation, and consumption of local, healthy, and culturally relevant food.

J. J. Lupinacci (✉)
Washington State University, Pullman, WA, USA

A. Happel-Parkins
University of Memphis, Memphis, TN, USA

© The Author(s) 2018                                                              91
S. Rice, A. G. Rud (eds.), *Educational Dimensions of School Lunch*,
https://doi.org/10.1007/978-3-319-72517-8_6

In the United States essentially all students have participated in the daily ritual of school lunch. Whether we brought our lunches from home or purchased a hot lunch from the cafeteria, school lunch played a huge part in our school experiences. However, for many children in the United States the National School Lunch Program (NSLP) provides essential sustenance for their development. In some cases, the NSLP may provide the *only* full meal students receive in a day. School food has recently been gaining attention from politicians, applauding or criticizing the Obama administration, which sought to implement standards that would increase nutritional value in meals provided by schools through the Healthy, Hunger-Free Kids Act (USDA 2017b, c; NEA 2017). However, federal attention on school lunches in the United States is not new to the politics of public schooling (Avey 2015). Stemming back to 1946 when US President Harry S. Truman signed the National School Lunch Act, school lunch provisions were made official by the 79th Congress. Senator Richard B. Russell Jr. (1946/2014) wrote in the act:

> It is hereby declared to be the policy of Congress, as a measure of national security, to safeguard the health and well-being of the Nation's children and to encourage the domestic consumption of nutritious agricultural commodities and other food, by assisting the States, through grants-in aid and other means, in providing an adequate supply of food and other facilities for the establishment, maintenance, operation and expansion of nonprofit school lunch programs. (Sec. 2 [42 U.S.C. 175], pp. 1–2)

Recently, the US government has rolled back the standards of the Healthy, Hunger-Free Kids Act, arguing that nutritious food is too expensive and often wasted by students. Secretary of Agriculture Sonny Perdue (USDA 2017a) announced the rolling back of standards on school food provided by the Healthy, Hunger-Free Kids Act in favor of providing "local flexibilities" for schools in regards to requirements for whole grains, sodium, and milk. Perdue explained, "If kids aren't eating the food, and it's ending up in the trash, they aren't getting any nutrition—thus undermining the intent of the program" (para. 2). School food is a political issue, a matter of national security, as well as a fundamental human right afforded to all by the Universal Declaration of Human Rights. While political agendas change, the importance of providing children with healthy, nourishing, and culturally appropriate food remains an important issue.

Writing about school food and the importance of learning about nutrition policy, Mary McKenna and Sharon Brodovsky (2016) acknowledged that students have questions about nutritional changes in school food. They explained that students ask questions such as:

> Why did my school stop selling chocolate chip cookies the size of my head? Why does not my school sell pop anymore? Why does all the pizza come with a whole-wheat crust? Why is there so much local food at school now? (p. 201)

McKenna and Brodovsky (2016) observed: "If students studied food and nutrition policies, they could answer these questions" (p. 201). Along with McKenna and Brodovsky, we take the position that learning *with* and *about* food as part of an engaged civic education is as important to national security and public health as serving healthy food for students to consume. In other words, we assert that providing children with healthy food needs to be accompanied with a curriculum that teaches children about the importance of local, healthy, and culturally appropriate foods. If it is true that students are throwing away copious amounts of school food—as some politicians maintain to justify the denial of healthy meals for students, despite research to the contrary from pediatricians (Johnson et al. 2016)—then a strong effort to educate young eaters about the importance of lifelong healthy eating habits is needed. However, this is no easy task and so in this chapter we turn to a case study to learn how a local food movement in Detroit works through local food policies to ensure healthy and culturally appropriate nourishment in schools, families, and communities.

When faced with the monumental challenges posed by an industrial food system, we turn to the generative process of sharing narratives, which we see as a critical praxis and cultural work. Drawing from Giroux (1992), Niewolny and D'Adamo-Damery (2016) defined cultural work "as moments of learning [that] provides us with a useful lens to help us navigate the epistemological and ontological conditions that inform our practices of resistance and change in alternative food system circles" (p. 114). Sharing narratives about community food work in the southern USA, these authors utilized stories as a way to "humanize the 'wicked problem' of food insecurity while creating new possibilities in our everyday work of resistance and learning" (p. 115). Many educators are faced with a growing number of students living in poverty and the consequent challenge of how they can best support all students in classrooms and communities. These conditions call for educators to ethically and critically question what it means to be educated. Included in this kind of questioning is the need to recognize *what is* and to rethink *what ought to be* taught in schools. Such questions become a catalyst for departures from modern conceptions of schooling and engage educators—especially school leaders and teacher educators—in learning from diverse traditions that not only broaden definitions of success in schools and society, but also strengthen the potential for communities to become spaces where people live equitably and sustainably.

Calling for educational researchers to take school food more seriously, Weaver-Hightower (2011) asserted, "Food is a basic aspect of life, intimately tied to our survival, our sense of self, our beliefs, our connection to or disconnection from others, and our impact on the natural world" (p. 15). While much could be said about the ways in which school food programs could provide more nutritious food to all students—as well as the importance of appropriate nutrition for childhood development and legislative efforts establishing what constitutes a healthy meal—we want to zoom further out and suggest that food, and thus meals like breakfast, lunch, and dinner are deeply political and cultural activities. Positioning school food within the broader cultural framework of community food, we argue for moving food practices from the hidden curriculum—or "the unwritten, unofficial, and often unintended lessons, values, and perspectives that students learn in school" (Abbott 2014, para. 1)—to a more explicit and critical role within the classroom. Following Weaver-Hightower's (2011) call for greater attention on the role of food in schools, we assert that educators and educational researchers need to work toward rethinking how it is we recognize and come to understand what we know about food. Accordingly, we ask: How can curriculum center on working together to learn from and with food movements while taking into account the policy, access, production, preparation, nutrition, and cultural relevancies of food?

## FOOD, SOCIAL JUSTICE, AND LEARNING TO LIVE WELL IN THE TWENTY-FIRST CENTURY

In the twenty-first century, we have already seen new challenges posed by rapidly changing climate systems and the unsustainable depletion of renewable and non-renewable resources. The increased connections between violent conflict and poverty with famine, drought, floods, earthquakes, and severe storms further contribute to massive income disparities and a growing number of families living in poverty (IPCC 2015). In the face of these issues, educators determined to make a difference have found hope in we refer to in this chapter as *the commons* and the valuable lessons learned from turning our attention toward the local and nurturing grass-roots wisdom shared by neighbors as they survive in difficult conditions. Despite the challenges of this century, diverse communities throughout the world are alive and rich with the daily practices of reciprocity and mutual aid. However, it is up to educators to facilitate student learning that is centered on experiences that reach outside the confines of an increasingly standardized Western industrial curriculum. This exploration of community beyond the strict confines of the standardized curriculum offers a plethora of opportunities for local-living community collabora-tions. These collaborations utilize an approach that we refer to as learning to "recognize, resist, and reconstitute" (Lupinacci and Happel-Parkins 2015) how we think and behave in our relationships to one another, our-selves, and the living systems within which we exist.

In our practice we draw from our experiences as scholar-activist researchers—from Alison's community activism and partnership with local food organizations and from Johnny as a school teacher and community activist in Detroit. While we do not specify precisely what should be taught in the twenty-first century, it has become clear to us that schooling—as it is commonly understood and practiced today—ought to be resisted and rethought. An economically centered globalizing institution that regularly employs a monocultured curriculum (Illich and Verne 1976; Spring 2015), Western industrial schooling is rooted in assumptions about educa-tion that work to undermine cultural and biological diversity across the globe. Whenever we are asked how we, as scholar-activist educators in such authoritarian times, might begin to teach in support of the commons and for equity among all relationships, we suggest that educators work to learn from the wisdom of grassroots women and men with a focus on something we all have in common—such as food, water, land, and air. Such a shift in the source of knowing offers tremendous hope shared through stories of resistance to the colonialism of Western industrial edu-cation and development.

Many of the challenges of today's dominant society are institutional-ized into schooling and thus are passed on to future generations via for-malized education. However, the power and influence that is vested in schools also allows for liberatory possibilities. In other words, what is taught has the potential to transform schools into valued public spaces that can work to deconstruct modern assumptions threatening equity among all beings in diverse living systems. Such possibilities require that educators commit to recognizing and attending to the everyday practices that support living in peace with each other and the more-than-human world. Furthermore, educators must recognize schools as potential sites of liberation and teach toward mutually sustaining and respectful relationships with an emphasis on aspects of the commons—such as food practices—that support local-living communities. A commitment to this perspective helps us to understand why we ought to rethink the role of education and where we as teachers and researchers might make a difference.

Drawing from the field of EcoJustice Education, we frame our work with a focus on diversity, democracy, and sustainability toward communities within which all human beings live with respect for one another and the planet's diverse living systems (Martusewicz et al. 2015; Lupinacci and Happel-Parkins 2015). This may sound a bit romantic and oversimplified; however, we are more and more convinced that it is precisely such optimism that allows for critical and ethical educators to refocus curriculum and pedagogy on identifying and recovering from destructive cultural habits by learning from wise members of our community who are living in sustainable ways. These members can help us learn how to live together equitably in a community and it is important to recognize that sometimes those wise members are not human beings (Lupinacci and Happel-Parkins 2017). This approach requires that we relocate knowledge and learning. Simply stated, we must expand our understandings of education in order to (re)value the local relationships that exist in our own neighborhoods where local peoples' traditions and wisdom can be valued and shared through common experiences and reciprocal relationships. Such an approach to rethinking schools and education incorporates lessons of generosity, food, and traditions that feed both the body and the mind. Unfortunately, many Western *educated* people have lost this knowledge.

## ENCLOSURES OF FOOD COMMONS

Drawing from the work of C.A. Bowers (2006, 2017), there are two important concepts that inform how we refer to food systems in this chapter. The first is *the commons*. As defined by Martusewicz et al. (2011), the commons are the "non-monetized relationships, practices and traditions that people across the world use to survive and take care of one another on a day-to-day basis" (p. 247). Martusewicz et al. identify two distinct spheres within the commons: *the cultural commons*—the practices, skills, and knowledge systems among people—and *the environmental commons*—the air, water, land, seeds, forests, and so on. In the EcoJustice Dictionary Bowers (2017) defined the commons as representing:

> both the naturals systems (water, air, soil, forests, oceans, etc.) and the cultural patterns and traditions (intergenerational knowledge ranging from growing and preparing food, medicinal practices, arts, crafts, ceremonies, etc.) that are shared without cost by all members of the community. (para. 1)

Conceptualizing the commons in this way illuminates the many ways in which aspects of diverse cultures and the environment are enclosed through privatization, commodification, colonization, and modernization. Calling attention to the concept of enclosure in relation to food, Martusewicz et al. (2011) explained, "Unless we grow our own food and husband the animals needed to provide meat, most of our food is provided through grocery stores that acquire food from around the world via a handful of huge privately owned multinational corporations" (p. 214).

Food enclosures refer to the socio-political and economic efforts to enclose and thus limit access to production, preparation, and consumption of local, healthy, and culturally relevant food. For example, affordable healthy food is often expensive and may only be available—if at all—through specialty grocery stores, markets, or big-box stores that can be difficult for marginalized populations to access. Another example of a condition resulting from food enclosures is the existence of *food deserts*—geographic locations without access to healthy food (Guthman 2011). Community members living within food deserts have little or no access to nourishing food and educational settings that promote food traditions to support physical and cultural health. Often lacking grocery stores, food deserts are geographic locations wherein most people can only access food at fast food restaurants, dollar stores, gas stations, liquor stores, and so on. As part of a larger unjust food distribution system, these types of food establishments are part of a broader distribution system primarily interested in profit and with little interest in or knowledge of local health. In a food desert, processed pre-packaged food—often laden with preservatives and processed sugars—are directly contributing to the failing health of many of the nation's vulnerable populations.

We assert that school food systems are often full of unhealthy food and harmful food practices for children, and that these conditions are a result of food enclosures. In other words, we assert that food crises are a result of a cultural crisis and the result of a fundamental flaw in how we understand—if we learn at all—the survival imperative of food as part of the commons. Highlighting the importance of the commons as diverse non-monetized aspects of local culture and of local environments, in this chapter we urge educators to consider how food enclosures can be understood and challenged through the recognition of damaging patterns in the daily actions and habits in classrooms. To that end, we share ecocritical lessons learned from the Detroit food movement that challenge us to recognize the importance of both learning that food is a right for all as well as the ways in which we can teach and learn with our students from, and through, radical food policy and activism.

## EVERYBODY NEEDS TO EAT: HUNGER, FOOD SECURITY, AND HUMAN RIGHTS

[We are fighting for] a world where...all peoples, nations and states are able to determine their own food producing systems and policies that provide every one of us with good quality, adequate, affordable, healthy, and culturally appropriate food. (Nyéléni 2007, p. 2)

How far away from healthy food are you? Do you have access to or knowledge of culturally relevant, affordable food ingredients and traditions? Most likely, if you are not low-income or living in a predominantly low-income neighborhood, then you have access to healthy food choices several times a day. However, if you happen to live in communities like so many urban and rural communities in the United States—you likely live in what is referred to as a food desert (Guthman 2011).

According to the Centers for Disease Control and Prevention (CDC), "Good nutrition can help lower risk for many chronic diseases, including heart disease, stroke, some cancers, diabetes, and osteoporosis" (CDC 2009, p. 7). Further, the CDC (2009) reported, "Health disparities in chronic disease incidence and mortality are widespread among members of racial and ethnic minority populations" (p. 1). Research linking nutrition to physical and mental health has found that malnourishment among adults and children is especially prevalent within vulnerable populations (CDC 2009; Seligman et al. 2011). Food options and choices have both short- and long-term health implication which are inextricably linked with systems of racism, classism, and sexism.

As diverse food traditions rapidly assimilate to Western industrial culture, there is an associated loss of the health and healing wisdom of the elders in our communities. While dominant discussions on food justice, hunger, and health are often informed by discourses of food security, a stronger and more sustainable discourse for addressing food justice is the concept of sovereignty—specifically what activists and the International Peasant's Movement, *La Via Campesina*, call *food sovereignty* (Nyéléni 2007). In the village of Nyéléni in Sélingué, Mali, in 2007, over 500 representatives of diverse grassroots organizations met in response to the growing experiences of local "capacities to produce healthy, good and abundant food...being threatened and undermined by neo-liberalism and global capitalism" (Nyéléni 2007, p. 1). Recognizing collective wisdom and self-determination of the world's women and indigenous cultures, they identified food sovereignty as having the "power to preserve, recover and build on our food producing knowledge and capacity" (Nyéléni 2007, p. 1). While this particular gathering was not the first of its kind, the participants produced The Declaration of Nyéléni (2007) within which they provide a succinct and widely used definition for food sovereignty. Nyéléni (2007)—the collective name decided upon by the group in honor of a legendary Malian woman who fed her people—define food sovereignty as "the right of peoples to healthy and culturally appropriate food produced through ecologically sound and sustainable methods, and their right to define their own food and agriculture systems" (p. 1).

Building from the valuable information and language that food security research and policy has to offer, this chapter explores how a very intentional group of local activists organize and subvert oppressive social, economic, and political systems. These activists are working to transform neighborhoods in Detroit from food deserts dependent on imported, unhealthy, cheap food into sovereign food systems with culturally relevant, nutritious, and affordable access to food. For the activist farmers in Detroit, in solidarity with *campesinos/as* around the world, the question became: How do we learn to prepare and grow culturally relevant and healthy food for ourselves?

Food ought to be what keeps us alive and connected to our diverse cultures and bioregions in ways that truly support diversity on the planet. However, as illuminated by the examples of the conditions in Detroit and Mali, the increased incidence of food insecurity is a pressing reality for many people living in the United States and the world (Coleman-Jensen et al. 2012; FAO et al. 2012). According to a study conducted in Detroit, Michigan, more than half a million Detroit residents live in areas defined as food deserts (MG Research and Consulting 2007). People in Detroit suffer from a lack of access to healthy, fresh food. This post-industrial phenomenon has created populations of people statistically more likely to suffer or die early deaths from diet-related disease than people who have access to healthy food. Referring to the Detroit study, Malik Yakini, a leader, activist, and educator in the Detroit Black Community Food Security Network (DBCFSN), explained:

> Researcher Mari Gallegher came to Detroit…and characterized much of Detroit as a food desert. An area, according to her definition, where Detroiters have to travel twice as far to get to a major grocer as they do to what she called a fringe food location or what we in Detroit call a party store—a store that sells alcohol, cigarettes, tobacco, potato chips, candy, and other things that can only nominally be considered to be food. (Yakini 2011)

Yakini continued to explain the work he does in the DBCFSN Network:

> Rather than just complain or lament about our condition, our organization practices self-determination. We think it is important that people themselves stand up and find solutions to our problems. One of the solutions to the lack of access to fresh affordable healthy produce in the city of Detroit is urban agriculture. (Yakini 2011)

While the damage caused by food deserts in Detroit is certainly devastating to the local community, as Yakini explained, there is a growing movement of resistance to this precarious reality. Local groups are responding to the lack of access to healthy food in Detroit by producing their own food and educating the youth on local food production. Such efforts to establish food sovereignty in Detroit have made significant gains through arguing food security as a fundamental human right.

## Food Is a Human Right

For over 60 years, international activists, politicians, and policy makers have used a human rights framework to take a legal, political, and cultural approach to recognizing food as a basic human right. The human right to adequate food falls under a broader human rights framework that ensures an adequate standard of living. Access to food and nutrition is often considered an economic right and thus nested within rights to wages, health, and a clean environment. The DBCFSN addresses these issues through a political discourse that advocates for a food secure city. However, before looking closely at the DBCFSN, it is important to understand the larger international context within which food security has come to be a human rights issue.

The drafting of the Universal Declaration of Human Rights (UDHR) in 1948 clearly outlined the importance of access to food for all people. Article 25 of the UDHR stated:

> Everyone has the right to a standard of living adequate for the health and well-being of himself or his family, including food, clothing, housing and medical care and necessary social services, and the right to security in the event of unemployment, sickness, disability, widowhood, old age or other lack of livelihood in circumstances beyond his control. (United Nations 1948, para. 1)

This was reinforced and further detailed in 1966 by Article 11 of the International Covenant on Economic, Social and Cultural Rights (ICESCR):

> The States Parties to the present Covenant recognize the right of everyone to an adequate standard of living for himself and his family [sic], including adequate food, clothing and housing, and to the continuous improvement of living conditions. (United Nations 1966, para. 1)

A decent standard of living is considered to be dependent on the security of individuals, or groups of individuals, as a fulfillment of civil liberties and freedom. A consistent trend in the world, especially in so-called developing countries, shows that those denied civil liberties suffer disproportionately from social injustice and severe deprivations (FAO et al. 2012). Included in this suffering are food insecurity, hunger-related disease, malnutrition, and preventable childhood mortality. Internationally, while hunger is still considered a world problem, food security and the right to food has been broadly embraced. Despite the international recognition of hunger, the United States has failed to recognize this basic human right. Currently, 162 countries have signed and ratified the covenant. As a legally binding agreement of international obligation to ratifying states, the ratification of this treaty commits a nation to implementing and enforcing the ICESCR. The United States is one of seven countries in the world that has signed but not yet ratified the ICESCR.

Unfortunately, the ICESCR and the UDHR alone fail to specifically address the human rights and unique needs of children. In 1989 the Convention on the Rights of the Child (CRC) was proposed to address this issue. In Article 24 the CRC stated:

> Children have the right to good quality health care—the best health care possible—to safe drinking water, nutritious food, a clean and safe environment, and information to help them stay healthy. Rich countries should help poorer countries achieve this. (United Nations 1989)

The CRC is one of the most widely accepted international agreements in the human rights framework with 193 state parties ratifying. Only the United States and Somalia have not yet ratified the CRC.

Despite the work of food advocacy groups and international governments trying to adhere to the treaty agreements of the UDHR, food and nutrition rights are often afterthoughts to perceived larger issues of human rights. Attention to hunger concerns, as one of the many human rights violations that impact low-income and marginalized populations, is one reason to argue for a human rights approach to food security. However, in the United States a systematic dismantling of the social safety net—including social security—has increased human rights violations and transformed a war against poverty into a war against poor people and thus poor children.

## HUNGER AND FOOD SECURITY IN THE UNITED STATES

It is disgraceful that in one of the world's most wealthy countries, hunger and malnutrition plague the daily lives of people in the United States. The most profound aspect of this human rights violation is that it is primarily an act of violence against children. According to the U.S. Department of Agriculture (USDA), in 2012 there were 33.1 million adults and 15.9 million children—or approximately 22% of all children in the United States—living in food insecure households (Coleman-Jensen et al. 2013). In addition to the 49 million living in food insecure homes, 7 million households were considered to have one or more persons suffering from hunger due to not being able to afford food despite food welfare programs.

The number of people denied access to food in the United States has grown from 13.5% of households that were food insecure in 1998 to 15.9% of households in 2012 (Coleman-Jensen et al. 2013). As a result of growing financial hardships and the recent national recession, the number of people living with hunger and limited access to food is increasing. Simply put, access to healthy food is an undeniable and crucial issue in the United States.

In the United States, food insecurity refers to being unable to obtain sufficient food for oneself or one's household (USDA 2016). People in this position must skip meals or cut back on the quality or quantity of food. In many developing countries around the world, famine and thus hunger is apparent and visible. However, in the United States, hunger is routinely obfuscated because folks in food deserts have abundant access to inexpensive yet unhealthy food. While starvation rarely occurs in the United States, children and adults frequently go hungry and a mild but consistent form of malnutrition occurs, causing long-term damage to adults and children (Krugman 2008). Despite the presence of government aid programs in the form of welfare food assistance, hunger and malnutrition most often occur in families who are classified as working poor. Drawing from U.S. Bureau of Labor Statistics (2016) data, the Center for Poverty Research at University of California State, Davis (2017) estimated that "about 9.5 million of people who spent at least 27 weeks in the labor force were poor" (para. 1.)

In the United States, issues of social welfare, like food security, do not go entirely unaddressed. However, with ongoing cutbacks to welfare programs, assistance to support the healthy development of healthy food secure households is inadequate and increasingly problematic. Restricted access to welfare and/or limits placed on welfare entitlements most severely impact children living in poverty. Welfare reform in the United States, under the misleading title of the Personal Responsibility and Work Opportunity Reconciliation Act (PRWORA), ties welfare entitlements such as food, childcare, and housing assistance to strict and inflexible work requirements and has systematically contributed to an increase in the number of children living in food insecure households.

One of the most vital supports for families living in conditions of poverty is food welfare assistance, or in what in the United States is called the Supplemental Nutrition Assistance Program (SNAP). Food welfare assistance enables poor families to receive government aid that they can use to purchase food. Unfortunately due to funding cuts and entitlement caps, it has become increasingly difficult in the United States to apply for and receive such food assistance. Decades of policy reform that has deregulated social responsibility for both federal and state governments has increased food insecurity for families. In Detroit, Michigan, only 8% of the recorded use of food welfare assistance was documented to be used at food retailers that provide healthy fresh food options (MG Research and Consulting 2007).

## RECOGNIZING AND RESISTING FOOD INSECURITY: THE BLACK COMMUNITY FOOD SECURITY NETWORK

A food desert in the United States is a visible phenomenon that exposes the intense levels of economic and racial inequality that exist beyond the deteriorating welfare system and encompasses overall food security. The damage caused by food deserts in Detroit has been endured by the city's residents since the beginning of deindustrialization. However, as mentioned earlier, local groups of activists and farmers are responding to the lack of healthy food in Detroit by producing their own food. Urban farms and local gardens are being established, revived, and maintained across throughout the city. As a major part of the work for strong food security, the food sovereignty movement has become a key influence and a growing source of inspiration.

DBCFSN is a food sovereignty group that has taken issue with the level of food insecurity in Detroit. They described the condition of living in a food desert as an act of aggression on racial and class minorities. The DBCFSN is a coalition of local activists who work together to counter the injustices of food insecurity by advocating and acting for strong food secure systems in Detroit. The DBCFSN was founded in February of 2006 with the specific intent to organize members of the community to play a more active role in establishing local food security. Recognizing food security as a crucial element in childhood health, well-being, and development, the network grew out of a local emphasis on food as a human right often denied to the Black community under the political structures of White supremacy. The DBCFSN is an African-centered learning community of food activists and producers that "works to build self-reliance, food security and justice in Detroit's Black community by influencing public policy, engaging in urban agriculture, promoting healthy eating, encouraging cooperative buying and directing youth towards careers in food-related fields" (DBCFSN 2016a, para. 1). The DBCFSN's (2016a) vision statement explains: "DBCFSN's vision is to advance movement towards food sovereignty while advocating for justice in the food system that ensures access to healthy foods with dignity and respect for all of Detroit's residents" (para. 1). Throughout this work, the DBCFSN emphasizes the importance of education—and specifically in developing a sense of agency in youth (DBCFSN 2016b)—in the process of working toward food sovereignty.

## A Case Study from Detroit: Urban Agriculture and Culturally Relevant Urban Education

In 2006 the DBCFSN took direct agricultural action in response to food insecurity by involving a local school in the short-term use of a quarter-acre plot on Detroit's east side. They planted and harvested vegetables and herbs and farmed on a community work schedule that included students, teachers, and parents from the community as well as local urban farmers. Unfortunately, they were forced to move after one year of successful farming when the city sold the land to a developer. In 2007, they continued the mission on a half-acre land on the city's west side. They named this the "D-town farm," which was a garden site for which the DBCFSN organized gardening beds and an irrigation system, cultivated local farming leaders, and sold produce locally in the neighborhood and at the city's farmer's market. One year later, with support from a strong policy proposal they drafted, the DBCFSN acquired a two-acre plot of land from the city. The plot was formerly a tree nursery and was located in a large city park. They negotiated an official agreement of usage of the land for a fixed fee of one dollar a year for ten years. Following the first two agricultural projects, "D-town farm" became an agricultural project that had grown in scale, decreasing local suffering from food insecurity. By 2009, the DBCFSN had expanded the number of local markets to which they provided fresh produce and began talks with the Detroit Public Schools in efforts to become a direct source of local healthy food for children (M. Yakini, personal communication, March 26, 2009).

This is an extremely important and a successful food sovereignty work. In a short span of time the agricultural projects of DBCFSN have become a primary source of food for local neighborhood people while directly involving local citizens in the food production process. Their effort to farm in Detroit is a political action taken to restore human dignity and make up for a complete disregard for the basic human right of access to healthy food. A strong aspect of the DBCFSN is their recognition of food insecurity as a problem that runs deeper than simply a lack of fresh and healthy food in the city. Their intersectional approach to understanding systemic food insecurity recognizes how racism, sexism, and classism all influence various aspects of people's lives—including the lack of access to transportation, an ineffective and almost non-existent public transportation system, a record high rate of unemployment, unsafe neighborhood conditions, and so on. These factors all directly impact Detroit citizens' right to access affordable and healthy food. The DBCFSN initiates work that feeds people and engages them in sustainable farming. Their work also emphasizes the importance of utilizing culturally relevant food practices that will continue to provide sustenance toward a healthier Detroit. Additionally, the DBCFSN recognizes the importance of ensuring that their food sovereignty efforts are supported by the local government.

## DETROIT FOOD SECURITY POLICY

In 2006, the DBCFSN went before the Neighborhood and Community Service Standing Committee of the Detroit City Council. The issue they brought before the City Council was the lack of comprehensive food security policy and the need to develop and implement such a policy. The DBCFSN was then appointed by the City of Detroit to draft and present such a policy. Over the following year the DBCFSN researched and wrote a food security policy for the city of Detroit. The DBCFSN recognized this as a serious opportunity and sought to form a committee specifically dedicated to this massive undertaking. The Public Policy Committee, a division of the DBCFSN, involved the community in this endeavor and held several public meetings from which they harvested feedback from local and international experts. The committee involved Dr. Kami Pothukuchi, from the Department of Urban Studies and Planning at Wayne State University, and included several recommendations from the committee's research in their presentation to the City Council. The Detroit City Council put the policy to a vote for approval and it unanimously passed. Detroit officially adopted a food security policy in March 2008. With official policy in place, the DBCFSN's battle for food security has been guaranteed a voice in the local government.

The success of local government's acknowledgment of food insecurity assisted the DBCFSN's political agenda and carved out a place at the decision-making table for other local organizations. In a relatively short amount of time the DBCFSN has engaged local citizens, policy makers, and community organizations in collaborating to ensure a food secure city. The result was a turning point, as public officials could now turn to local organizations for input and assistance on the issue of hunger in Detroit rather than solely relying on assistance from outside experts. As a result of these efforts the Detroit Food Security Policy (DFSP) was born. The DFSP served as a catalyst for a political alliance between over 30 of the city's most active organizations concerned with long-term social justice and sustainability in Detroit. This is truly a unique and powerful alliance as many of these organizations are often forced into competition with each other for limited resources and funding. Yet, they find themselves unified by shared interests and the food sovereignty movement stewarded by the DBCFSN. Under the umbrella of a shared goal of food security, they collectively have a stronger voice in the political process.

The political agenda and policy initiatives of the DBCFSN embedded within the DFSP have created a massive opportunity for Detroit to reclaim food security. The DFSP reflects much of the vision of the DBCFSN, but most important to the movement is the focus on education which the organization has retained since its inception. The DFSP strongly emphasizes the importance of education in playing a role in establishing food security. The document recognizes that providing healthy food is only one step toward food security. Education is a central component of food security, as healthy, food-conscious citizens who know and are free to make healthy choices in regards to food production and consumption must be cultivated. The approach to education called for in the DFSP directly addresses the cultural habits that undermine social justice and sustainability for all members of the local community and are directly connected to the quality of public education. Simply put, the DFSP helps to provide policy that creates the opportunity for a serious conversation about how educational reform might better support children learning in all neighborhoods in the city while highlighting that any significant reform must work toward the creation of a healthy, equal, and culturally responsive education for all children. For any community that does not know how to access, grow, and prepare healthy food, food security is merely an idea rather than a reality. Without education, the agricultural efforts of the DBCFSN are reduced to short-term aid for the hungry and are not likely to be sustained.

Recognizing this, the DBCFSN advocates for citizens to engage in learning important connections between food and health issues in the community. They advocate for and practice a strong belief that citizens should have access to affordable healthy food as well as to education that exposes the conditions under which food insecurity is created and maintained in poor communities.

The DBCFSN has implemented school reform that has reached public schools, public and private charter schools, churches, community organizations, shelters, hospitals, and many before- and after-school programs in Detroit. In all cases, a focal point of this local reform is the consideration of educational impact on the dietary habits and health of the local community. The DBCFSN recognizes the potential impact that can be made by educational reform that purposefully aims to foster and develop learning opportunities for members of the community. These opportunities address community members' rights to a happy and healthy life as well as how they can actively work to provide such a life for themselves, their children, and their grandchildren. The DBCFSN also recognizes that as sites of learning, schools ought to be places that offer healthful food. This interest in healthy school food was taken up nationally by former First Lady Michelle Obama in her "Let's Move" campaign to end childhood obesity (http://www.letsmove.gov/) and other initiatives, such as Healthy, Hunger-Free Kids Act of 2010, to fund childhood nutrition and free healthy lunch programs. In Detroit, the DBCFSN and the DFSP provided a solid model for how to work with schools and organizations to provide educational reform that teaches the community to be leaders in both establishing local food security and becoming the suppliers of the local healthy food.

From the case of the DBCFSN we can learn how a food sovereignty movement can benefit from engaging in political work framed in a food security discourse to begin to shift that discourse to one more centered on food sovereignty. Schools across the nation have perpetuated several bad food practices ranging from candy sales to the serving of horrifying meals consisting of processed foods—almost always laden with excessive amounts of processed sugar—that have little or no long-term nutritional value (Cordain et al. 2005; Monteiro 2009). The DBCFSN works to establish the right for all children in Detroit to attend schools that plant, tend, and harvest food as part of the school's curriculum. The schools that they have partnered with have become a neighborhood food source wherein the community, especially the children, convenes to learn to eat and prepare locally cultivated, culturally appropriate, healthy, and affordable food.

## LEARNING FROM DETROIT: LOCAL WISDOM
## AND A MOVEMENT TO LOCALIZE FOOD

In the context of recognizing and reconnecting with our commons, and common sense, in efforts to better support *all* students, we find Detroit—like so many other communities around the world for which modern economics has failed—to be rich with hope and promise despite the clearly visible economic abandonment and worldwide notoriety for violence and crime. Despite the constant depiction of Detroit as a place of abandonment and industrial failure, it is a place of great wealth in terms of resilience and determination.

The cultural assumptions that dominate perceptions of Detroit as a city of racialized poverty tell us that Detroit is a failure—an epic site of ruins to be rescued by tourism, development, and exploitation. Such assumptions are sadly similar to the ways in which many students living in poverty are perceived by schools. Education is often understood as the pathway for youth either to leave the city or to be trained to work in a low-wage economy with little or no social welfare. Such assumptions and perceptions play into sorting students into systemic poverty, military service, and/or seeking economic opportunity through informal economies that are illegal and thus tracking youth into prisons.

As a city that many consider the epitome for what happens when industry collapses and abandons the local, it is important that we learn from the ways Detroit is alive, growing, and resilient. We can learn from the diverse species as they grow from the land and aid in repopulating the ruins of factories, as diverse plant life and animals seeking new habitat overtake the concrete and metal. These efforts from both human and more-than-human beings, not only remind us of the living systems to which we belong but they also offer a strong example of how, beneath the layers of concrete and concepts of industrialization, efforts to strengthen and sustain life remain in abundance.

While this chapter is not intended to provide a generalized example, it draws from efforts in Detroit to share how an organization rooted in food sovereignty works through a human rights framework to create educational spaces devoted to initiating, developing, and sustaining the local commons through food sovereignty. In Detroit the food sovereignty movement provides the opportunity for leaders in the community—whether they be teachers, researchers, activists, pastors, or parents—to shift the current knowledge about and access to culturally appropriate and healthy food and respond to the systematic political and economic rationalization for not feeding our communities. In other words, there are activist-educators working in Detroit to feed students while simultaneously teaching students and families how to feed the community through reclaiming their rights to food and water. The message is simple; food is essential to the cultural and biological strength of any community and to systematically deny that right ought to be met with strong localized resistance. A fundamental position of educators supportive of equity for all students is that education can play a role in identifying and examining root causes of social suffering and environmental degradation. We have a collective responsibility to recognize the ways that we engage our students in how they learn to think and act in support of self-reliant food systems—and ultimately in local decision-making. Furthermore, if such local decision-making is the goal, then as educators we must understand and commit to empowering youth through fostering the development of a holistic curriculum that is culturally relevant and ecologically sustainable. Everybody eats and eating is an ethical relationship necessary for human survival. It seems logical, even commonsensical, that rethinking the purpose of education might include something as fundamental as knowledge of how to eat and preserve, or in some cases reclaim, the right to such life-sustaining traditions as growing food.

There are many recommendations that can be made for education that supports food sovereignty and thus address how we might best support students experiencing poverty. Schools should encourage young people toward an economic future in local agricultural practices that contribute to a direct reduction of dependency on outsiders who have systematically failed and continue to fail the local community. Working to structure curriculum around the vitality, or potential vitality, of the local community in partnership with schools exposes the politics of food while offering a solution, or even solutions, that simultaneously addresses local hunger, empowers students, and strengthens community.

Focusing on food and lessons learned from Detroit, some practical recommendations include eliminating foods and drinks with high sugar content, artificial preservatives, and artificial dyes from meals and from vending machines in schools. Furthermore, in doing so, educators can involve students in researching why such changes are being made as part of the curriculum. In this sense, students are not learning from top-down policy changes but rather they are actively taking part in the change. Since nutritious food is often systemically made inaccessible to children and families living in poverty, the curriculum of neighborhood schools can be refocused on reclaiming the food commons from food as a commodity controlled by corporations. If educators were to take seriously the revitalization of the commons and begin with food sovereignty in our communities, then every school should have a school garden, or farm. These sites could provide for healthy lunches that also serve as an experiential space for learning how to cultivate culturally appropriate and healthy food as a fundamental part of the curriculum.

In all cases, at the very least, school reform needs to commit to feeding children healthy food. Simultaneously, the curriculum ought to foster creativity, innovation, and ethics in rethinking farming and our food production practices to include appropriate technologies like rooftop gardening, aquaponics, hydroponics, and other potentially sustainable and equitable practices for growing and distributing healthy, culturally appropriate food. This both responds to the economic recession and creates opportunities for young people to become producers of local healthy food and contribute to an economy of scale based on mutual success rather than exploitation and exportation. In summary, the overall strategies we are suggesting require school leaders to push for policy reform and take actions toward directly feeding communities while supporting education that engages all students in such direct action empowerment. Detroit is a leader, among many other communities, in a worldwide yet localized food revolution that serves as a catalyst for a social movement that not only feeds Detroit but also can potentially feed the world.

## CONCLUSION: RETHINKING EDUCATION FOR AN ECOLOGICALLY JUST FUTURE

The more that educators engage in recognizing and reclaiming the local commons, the more potential there is for educational experiences that support teachers and students learning together to recognize the harmful assumptions and actions that undergird social and ecological injustice. In order to confront the growing inequity in schools, we argue it is most important to reframe how it is we understand the purpose of education. Asking questions like: (1) Does our curriculum support *all* students' health and well-being? (2) How is it we define success? and (3) What can we do to empower not only the students in our classroom but also future generations of students for hundreds of years to come? It is paramount that educators work as allies to those suffering while also challenging and confronting the systemic roots of oppression on our respective fronts. In other words, we all have a responsibility—many of us as privileged members of an unjust society—to support those suffering unjustly in whatever capacity we can.

In such authoritarian times, it is important that educators challenge dominant perceptions of what constitutes schooling, education, and knowledge to collectively imagine with open hearts and minds what is possible. Through a commons curriculum that focuses on reimagining our relationships with things we share in common—such as food, the air, water, and so on—we can teach toward a very different future for all students. Additionally, when we refocus curriculum on localized responses to issues directly impacting our communities, we challenge the prevalent individualism and isolation that is created through the neoliberal state. We learn through such curriculum to make friends with one another and to learn about, respect, and connect with those who produce and/or cultivate our food—be it local farmers, plants, a river, the food that we grow, or the soil that gives us life. It does not matter who or what exactly we befriend. The point is that we learn compassion, dependency, and different ways of listening and communicating when we understand in an ecological sense what it means to be friends—to recognize and value that we are in relationship with a vast variety of diverse beings and that we owe our existence to these relationships. Such a shift in education reclaims as part of the commons what it means to belong and contribute. In a commons curriculum, one in which we are suggesting to begin with food, we learn what it means to belong without fitting that understanding within a Western industrial framework. Rather, belonging becomes the relationships that we enact in our everyday lives, existing within healthy and mutually supportive ecosystems. It is through these friendly and interdependent relationships that we learn to overcome the isolating ills of Western industrial culture, and we are called to act with our diverse sisters and brothers to rethink not only how we best support children experiencing poverty but also how and what we teach all students.

## REFERENCES

Abbott, S. (2014). Hidden curriculum. *The glossary of education reform*. Retrieved from http://edglossary.org/hidden-curriculum

Avey, T. (2015). *The history of school lunch*. Public Broadcasting Network (PBS). Retrieved from http://www.pbs.org/food/the-history-kitchen/history-school-lunch/

Bowers, C. A. (2006). *Revitalizing the commons: Cultural and educational sites of resistance and affirmation*. Lanham: Lexington Books.

Bowers, C. A. (2017). Commons. In C. A. Bowers (Ed.), *The EcoJustice dictionary.* Retrieved from http://www.cabowers.net/dicterm/CAdict003.php

Center for Poverty Research. (2017). *Who are the working poor in America? Data from the Bureau of Labor Statistics.* Davis: University of California State. Retrieved from https://poverty.ucdavis.edu/faq/who-are-working-poor-america

Centers for Chronic Disease Control and Prevention (CDC). (2009). *The power of prevention chronic disease: The public health challenge of the 21st century.* Retrieved from http://www.cdc.gov/chronicdisease/pdf/2009-power-of-prevention.pdf

Coleman-Jensen, A., Nord, M., Andrews, M., & Carlson, S. (2012). *Household food security in the United States in 2011.* Washington, DC: United States Department of Agriculture (USDA).

Coleman-Jensen, A., Nord, M., & Singh, A. (2013). *Household food security in the United States in 2012.* Washington, DC: United States Department of Agriculture (USDA).

Cordain, L., Boyd Eaton, S., Sebastian, A., Mann, N., Lindeberg, S., Watkins, B. A., O'Keefe, J. H., & Brand-Miller, J. (2005). Origins and evolution of the Western diet: Health implications for the 21st century. *The American Journal of Clinical Nutrition, 81*(2), 341–335.

Detroit Black Community Food Security Network (DBCFSN). (2016a). *Our mission, vision, and values.* Detroit. Retrieved from https://detroitblackfoodsecurity.org/aboutus/vision-values1/#1481166384142-8e585330-bbae

Detroit Black Community Food Security Network (DBCFSN). (2016b). *Educational & youth programs.* Detroit. Retrieved from https://detroitblackfoodsecurity.org/educational-youth-programs/

FAO, WFP, & IFAD. (2012). *The state of food insecurity in the world 2012: Economic growth is necessary but not sufficient to accelerate reduction of hunger and malnutrition.* Rome: Food and Agriculture Organization of the United Nations (FAO).

Giroux, H. (1992). *Border crossings: Cultural workers and the politics of education.* New York: Routledge.

Guthman, J. (2011). *Weighing in: Obesity, food justice, and the limits of capitalism.* Berkeley: University of California Press.

Illich, I., & Verne, E. (1976). *Imprisoned in the global classroom.* New York: Writers and Readers.

Intergovernmental Panel on Climate Change (IPCC). (2015). *Climate change 2014: Synthesis report.* Geneva: IPCC. Retrieved from http://www.ipcc.ch/pdf/assessment-report/ar5/wg2/ar5_wgII_spm_en.pdf

Johnson, D. B., Podrabsky, M., Rocha, A., & Otten, J. J. (2016). Effect of the healthy hunger-free kids act on the nutritional quality of meals selected by students and school lunch participation rates. *JAMA Pediatrics.* Retrieved from http://jamanetwork.com/journals/jamapediatrics/fullarticle/2478057

114    J. J. LUPINACCI AND A. HAPPEL-PARKINS

Krugman, P. (2008, February 18). *Poverty is poison.* The New York Times. Retrieved from: http://www.nytimes.com/2008/02/18/opinion/18krugman.htm

Lupinacci, J., & Happel-Parkins, A. (2015). Recognize, resist, and reconstitute: An ecocritical framework in teacher education. *The SoJo Journal: Educational Foundations and Social Justice Education, 1*(1), 45–61.

Lupinacci, J., & Happel-Parkins, A. (2017). Ecocritically (re)considering STEM: Integrated ecological inquiry in teacher education. *Issues in Teacher Education, 26*(3), 52–64.

Martusewicz, R., Edmundson, J., & Lupinacci, J. (2011). *EcoJustice education: Toward diverse, democratic, and sustainable communities.* New York: Routledge.

Martusewicz, R., Edmundson, J., & Lupinacci, J. (2015). *EcoJustice education: Toward diverse, democratic, and sustainable communities* (2nd ed.). New York: Routledge.

McKenna, M., & Brodovsky, S. (2016). School food and nutrition policies as tools for learning. In J. Sumner (Ed.), *Learning, food, & sustainability: Sites for resistance and change* (pp. 201–220). New York: Palgrave.

MG Research & Consulting. (2007). *Examining the impact of food deserts on public health in Detroit.* Retrieved from http://marigallagher.com/projects/

Monteiro, C. A. (2009). Nutrition and health. The issue is not food, nor nutrients, so much as processing. *Public Health Nutrition, 12*(5), 729.

National Education Association (NEA). (2017). *Child nutrition.* Issues and action. Retrieved from http://www.nea.org/home/38649.htm

Niewolny, K. L., & D'Adamo-Damery, P. (2016). Learning through story as political praxis: The role of narratives in community food work. In J. Sumner (Ed.), *Learning, food, & sustainability: Sites for resistance and change* (pp. 113–132). New York: Palgrave.

Nyéléni. (2007). *Declaration of Nyéléni.* Sélingué: Nyéléni.

Russell, R. B. (2014). *Richard B. Russell national school lunch act.* U.S. Government. Retrieved from https://www.fns.usda.gov/sites/default/files/NSLA.pdf

Seligman, H. K., Laraia, B. A., & Kushel, M. B. (2011). Food insecurity is associated with chronic disease among low-income NHANES participants. *The Journal of Nutrition, 140*, 304–310.

Spring, J. (2015). *Globalization of education: An introduction.* New York: Routledge.

U.S. Bureau of Labor Statistics. (2016). *A profile of the working poor, 2014.* BLS report 1060. Retrieved from https://www.bls.gov/opub/reports/working-poor/2014/home.htm

U.S. Department of Agriculture (USDA). (2016). *Definitions of food security.* Economic Research Service. Retrieved from https://www.ers.usda.gov/topics/food-nutrition-assistance/food-security-in-the-us/definitions-of-food-security/

U.S. Department of Agriculture (USDA). (2017a). *Press release: Ag secretary Perdue moves to make school meals great again.* Press releases. Retrieved from https://www.usda.gov/media/press-releases/2017/05/01/ag-secretary-perdue-moves-make-school-meals-great-again

U.S. Department of Agriculture (USDA). (2017b). *Healthy hunger-free kids act.* Food and Nutrition Service. Retrieved from https://www.fns.usda.gov/tags/healthy-hunger-free-kids-act-0

U.S. Department of Agriculture (USDA). (2017c). *School meals: Healthy hunger-free kids act.* Food and Nutrition Service. Retrieved from https://www.fns.usda.gov/school-meals/healthy-hunger-free-kids-act

United Nations. (1948). *Universal declaration of human rights text of the declaration.* United Nations Publications. Retrieved from the United Nations website. http://www.un.org/en/documents/udhr/

United Nations. (1966). *International convention on economic, social, and cultural rights.* United Nations Publications. Retrieved from the Office of the United Nations High Commissioner for Human Rights website. http://www2.ohchr.org/english/law/pdf/cescr.pdf

United Nations. (1989). *Convention on the rights of the child. United Nations Publications.* Retrieved from the Office of the United Nations High Commissioner for Human Rights website. http://www2.ohchr.org/english/law/pdf/crc.pdf

Weaver-Hightower, M. B. (2011). Why education researchers should take school food seriously. *Educational Researcher, 40*(1), 15–21.

Yakini, M. [Sun Rhythms]. (2011, October 9). *System change – Malik Yakini* [Video file]. Retrieved from https://www.youtube.com/watch?v=NG3T3B0M0iE

# CHAPTER 7

# Education Toward an Increasingly Integrated Outlook on Meat

*Suzanne Rice*

Some students eat a brown bag meal they or their parents assemble at home. Others participate in the National School Lunch Program and eat whatever is on offer in the school cafeteria. A relatively small minority of students drive to a fast food eatery for a burger and fries or similar fare. Until a few decades ago, some students walked home for a noontime meal, but that practice has dwindled to near non-existence. Despite these and many other differences between students' lunchtime experiences, most have at least one thing in common: some kind of meat. It is estimated that 93 percent of youth aged 8 to 18 are meat-eaters (Stahler 2010), and at lunch, that part of the meal will likely be in the form of chicken nuggets, burgers, pizza toppings, or cold cuts.

As several authors in this volume observe, teachers, administrators, and students themselves generally treat school lunch as incidental to the real work of education. When any serious thought is given to school lunch, it is usually focused narrowly on the food actually consumed (most notably its taste or nutritional value). The food students actually consume during the lunch hour and throughout the day, while undeniably important, is but one "moment" of a complex phenomenon; the burger or nuggets eaten at lunchtime are parts of a food *system*—as are the students who eat them.

S. Rice (✉)
University of Kansas, Lawrence, KS, USA

© The Author(s) 2018
S. Rice, A. G. Rud (eds.), *Educational Dimensions of School Lunch*,
https://doi.org/10.1007/978-3-319-72517-8_7

This chapter adopts an intentionally educational stance toward school lunch, with "education" conceptualized along lines developed by Phillip Phenix. Above all, Phenix saw education as a process by which the typically unremarkable is made meaningful. In his words: "It is the office of education to widen one's view of life, to deepen insight into relationships, and to counteract the provincialism of customary existence—in short to engender an integrated outlook" (Phenix 1964, pp. 3–4). An integrated outlook is one in which each part of multifaceted phenomena is understood in terms of its bearing on one or more of the other parts and how these parts work together and comprise the whole. An integrated outlook is concerned with connections, relations, and interrelations. The learner is a part of the multifaceted phenomena he or she perceives, sometimes only as a perceiver and interpreter, but other times as a more obviously active participant. When a student considers such things as how the choice to either bike or drive to school affects not only travel time and cost, but also air quality, and, perhaps, how, in turn, air quality affects a classmate's asthma, he/she is in the process of developing a more integrated outlook, making connections between things that once appeared unrelated. The student is also exercising (and thereby likely strengthening) a moral inclination, that of taking another's welfare into consideration when making a decision that, to some observers, might seem to affect only self. The student begins to more fully grasp the range and depth of the connections between self and others.

Of central concern in this chapter is what might be entailed in helping students gain a more integrated outlook in respect of food, particularly food derived from other animals, consumed as part of school lunch and throughout the day. The focus here is on food derived from animals, rather than food in general, because most people, students and adults alike, are shielded from great swaths of knowledge about such food. For example, most do not know that, in the context of contemporary agricultural practices, the production of meat-based foods entails significant harm to the environment, to animals which become food, and to humans— those who eat certain kinds or quantities of animal-derived food or carry on animal agriculture. Some aspects of the knowledge at issue are literally kept at a distance. For example, animals destined for human consumption are fattened and slaughtered far away from large human population centers, where their sights, sounds, and smells are less likely to draw attention. The people employed in animal agriculture usually live near their work in relatively isolated rural communities and have few opportunities to directly share their experiences with outsiders; they may sign non-disclosure type agreements. In addition to physical distance, laws are also used to keep the public unaware of especially unsavory aspects of meat production. Access to slaughterhouses has always been controlled, but beginning in the 1990s, states began passing agricultural gag laws aimed at making it harder still for animal welfare advocates, environmentalists, and other investigators to witness and report what happens in and around these facilities (Pachirat 2011, pp. 133–150).

In various ways, relaxation, fun, and festivity also obscure harms embodied in the food students eat. Inside schools, meat-laden meals are part of the longest and typically most welcome break in students' days. This is a time when, at most schools, students can spend time with friends over a meal that will likely include such favorites as burgers, pizza, or chicken nuggets. For millions of students, this meal will be provided and thereby tacitly endorsed by the National School Lunch Program. Outside school, reassuring messages and emotionally positively charged activities connect meat eating with wholesomeness and happiness. On television, laughing cows promote cheese made from their milk and chatty tunas advertise the flesh of their bodies. Hotdogs are as much a part of the historical national pastime as home runs and as much a part of Independence Day as sparklers. At the major fast food restaurants, colorful toys and collectables are packaged alongside burgers and chicken nuggets. Nearly all of the widely celebrated holiday meals feature animal-based foods.

Most students are unaware or only vaguely aware of how the hamburger or chicken nugget enjoyed at lunchtime is connected to the environment and climate, to other-than-human-animals, and to the health of the eater himself or herself or to the workers who helped produce the burger or nugget. When students are unaware that the food they consume is related to phenomena and entities beyond the food itself, their capacity for engaging in the food system responsibly is significantly diminished. As students gain a more integrated outlook, they will begin to perceive connections and relations—between, for example, their burger or chicken patty and water pollution or the suffering of industrially farmed cows and chickens. Educating students about relations and connections involving food does not ensure any particular outcome, but it does provide students an opportunity to better understand the food system of which they are a part and, from there, to consider how they might best participate in, or perhaps even work to change, that system.

This chapter has two main parts. The first main part is divided into three sections. The first of these sections discusses environmental harms such as climate change and pollution, the second discusses animal suffering in the context of industrial farming, and the third discusses human health risks linked to animal agriculture and to the consumption of certain kinds or quantities of animal-based foods. The primary aim of these discussions is to provide information about aspects of meat production and consumption that is not in wide circulation among students—or adults. The second main part of the chapter discusses ways teachers might help students gain a more integrated outlook on the meat-based food they eat in the school lunchroom and throughout the day. The aim of this discussion is to provide a sense of the range of possible alternatives available rather than to recommend any specific course of action.

## SELDOM RECOGNIZED ASPECTS OF THE MEAT EATEN BY STUDENTS AND THE REST OF US

### The Environment and Climate

The burgers and nuggets students eat at lunchtime are made possible through practices that are harmful to the environment and climate. These practices center around concentrated animal feeding operations (CAFOs). Nearly all the animals destined to become food are now raised in CAFOs, also called industrial or factory farms, although the facilities are anything but bucolic (Hauter 2012; Leonard 2014). There were 4250 CAFOs in the United States in 2015 (U.S. Government Accountability Office 2016).

CAFOs are enormous facilities, each containing between thousands of larger animals, such as cows, and hundreds of thousands of smaller animals, such as chickens (Gurian-Sherman 2008, p. 2). CAFOs are designed for efficiency; these are the facilities where animals are grown as cheaply and quickly as possible. To that end, depending on species, animals are given special diets, typically containing a mixture of plant-based products, such as corn and soybeans, animal-based ingredients, such as rendered animal carcasses and animal waste products, and antibiotics and metals, such as organoarsenicals (Sapkota et al. 2007). Rendered animal products and waste are used as inexpensive sources of protein; antibiotics are included to suppress the spread of diseases and to promote growth; organoarsenicals (contained mostly in poultry feed) are used to promote growth. The impact of modern agriculture on the animals raised to become food, the climate and environment, and on human health is directly connected to what animals themselves are fed to begin with (Imhoff 2010; Kirby 2010; Lymbery 2014).

Industrial animal agriculture contributes to climate change by releasing an enormous volume of greenhouse gases into the atmosphere. Recent studies show that greenhouse gases resulting from livestock production are greater than those resulting from the entire transportation sector (United Nations Food and Agriculture Organization 2006, p. xxi; Pew Commission 2016). One of these gases is carbon dioxide, resulting mainly from deforestation, which occurs when land is cleared of native plants in order to grow feed crops, such as corn and soybeans. The planting, harvesting, and processing of corn, soybeans, and other plants used in animal feeds also require great quantities of carbon dioxide-emitting fertilizer and fossil fuel. There are still other carbon dioxide releasing events: animal feed is transported to CAFOs, fattened animals are trucked to slaughterhouses, meat and other animal parts are shipped to wholesalers and retailers (often overseas), and from there are driven to eating establishments and households.

Other greenhouse gases are worse than carbon dioxide for global warming potential (GWP). Methane, a gas produced during digestion, has 23 times the GWP of carbon dioxide. The billions of animals raised each year for food release 37 percent of the methane into the atmosphere. Nitrous oxide is another powerful greenhouse gas, with nearly 300 times the GWP of carbon dioxide. Industrial animal farming is responsible for 65 percent of the total nitrous oxide emissions, which come mainly from manure, but also from fertilizers, and fossil fuel combustion (United Nations Food and Agriculture Organization 2006, p. xxi; Pew Commission 2016).

The 27 billion animals raised in factory farms each year produce a huge volume of waste—1.3 billion tons a year—which is approximately 130 times more than that produced by humans (Solotaroff 2013; Castle and Goodman 2014). Untreated animal waste is commonly stored in massive "slurry lagoons," where it breeds bacteria. The bacteria, when combined with other airborne particles such as manure dust, forms nitric acid and returns to earth in the form of nitric acid rain, harming not only the soil, but also forest habitats and water ecosystems.

Local water supplies are polluted when animal waste leaks or is drained from slurry lagoons. Nitrogen and phosphorus from manure and fertilizer lead to the growth of algal blooms that deplete oxygen and asphyxiate fish

122    S. RICE

and other marine life. Toxic organisms in animal waste are also lethal (Hribar 2010, pp. 2–5). Millions of fish die when catastrophic lagoon failures spill "tens of millions of gallons" of untreated manure into waterways (Gurian-Sherman 2008, pp. 3–4). Industrial fish farming, which entails raising large numbers of fish in enclosures, creates tons of fecal waste that pollutes and deoxygenates aquatic habitats (Food Empowerment Project 2016).

Slaughterhouses are also a significant contributor to water pollution. Put together, US slaughterhouses pour over 50 million gallons of pollutants into waterways annually. Eight slaughterhouses are ranked among the top 20 surface water polluters in the country, emitting some 30 million pounds of contaminants each year. Slaughterhouse pollutants include blood, fat, manure, and other organic solids and various chemicals, including nitrogen, phosphorus, and ammonia (Farr 2015).

### Animals Raised to Become Food

The burgers and nuggets students eat at lunchtime were once sentient beings, and there is overwhelming evidence that animals used to make these and other meat-based foods endure varying degrees of fear, pain, and suffering, often over extended periods. Of course, at some point, animals used for food are deemed ready for "harvest," and their lives are terminated.[1] Among the general public, there is fairly widespread concern over the welfare of animals raised for human consumption, but even most adults seem to lack knowledge about the extent and depth of animal suffering entailed in the production of meat (Clark et al. 2016). Children's ignorance of this suffering is no doubt greater than that of adults.

While access to CAFOs is limited, journalists, environmentalists, and others have gathered evidence about the conditions in these facilities, and their accounts are deeply disturbing (Coe 1995; Eisnitz 2007; Foer 2009; Genoways 2014; Faruqi 2015; Solotaroff 2013). Typically, animals are kept in cages, stalls, and pens that are often so small that the creatures they contain are unable to turn their bodies or extend their legs or wings; sometimes animals are chained. Surgery without anesthetic is common in CAFOs: piglets' tails are "docked," chicks' beaks are seared or clipped, and cows' horns are sawed off or chemically shortened (Imhoff 2010, p. xv). Animal injuries and illnesses are also common in CAFOs. In these facilities, chickens, for example, reach a weight of five pounds in about 45 days; under normal circumstances, reaching that weight takes twice as long. The birds' legs often break under all that rapidly gained weight

(Castle and Goodman 2014, p. 10). Cows, confined together by the thousands, "stand knee deep in their own…[waste] covered in flies… [O]pen and festering sores on the cows' hides are left untreated" (Castle and Goodman, p. 11). In hog CAFOs, death by trampling is common because the animals are crammed into such small enclosures. Diseases from microbes, fungi, and parasites are a constant threat: "Accordingly, factory pigs are infused with a huge range of antibiotics and vaccines, and are doused with insecticides. Without these compounds – oxytetracycline, draxxin, ceftiofur, tiamulin – diseases would likely kill them. Thus factory-farm pigs remain in a state of dying until they're slaughtered" (Tietz 2006, n.p.). In CAFOs, most animals will experience no naturally occurring environmental stimuli and will never see sunlight, breathe fresh air, or set foot on grass or soil (Imhoff 2010, p. 3). The ammonia and hydrogen sulfide fumes from the urine and manure of thousands of animals burns these creatures' eyes and lungs and, in the absence of ventilation fans, would quickly reach lethal levels (Foer 2009, pp. 174–178).

Once fattened, animals destined to become food are transported to slaughterhouses where they are killed. There were 1100 slaughterhouses in the United States in 2015 (U.S. Government Accountability Office 2016, p. 5). Like CAFOs, slaughterhouses are largely shielded from observation. Nevertheless, accounts of slaughterhouse workers, undercover investigators, and others do see the light of day (Pachirat 2011; Eisnitz 2007). Such accounts reveal that, for many animals, the final minutes or hours of life are filled with terror and agony. It is not uncommon for animals to be bled, skinned (or scalded and plucked), and dismembered while they are still conscious (Pitney 2016; Foer 2009, pp. 226–233). In the United States, billions of land animals are killed for food each year. In 2014, this included 30 million cows, over 1 billion pigs, 2.5 billion turkeys, 2 million lambs and sheep, and nearly 9 billion chickens (Humane Society of the United States 2015).

## Implications for Human Health

The burgers and nuggets students eat at lunchtime have serious health implications, some of which are shared by all humans, and others of which are more localized, affecting particular groups. The health of all humans, regardless of whether they are meat eaters or vegans, is threatened by climate change, a process in which industrial animal agriculture is deeply implicated. As summarized in the 2014 National Climate Assessment:

"Climate change threatens human health and well-being in many ways, including impacts from increased extreme weather events, wildfire, decreased air quality, threats to mental health, and illnesses transmitted by food, water, and disease-carriers such as mosquitoes and ticks. Some of these health impacts are already underway in the United States." (Global Change Research Program 2014).

There are also health risks associated with eating the flesh of animals raised on industrial farms, including exposure to growth hormones and other chemicals widely used in commercially raised animals and exposure to Salmonella, Listeria, Campylobacter, Cryptosporidium, Giardia, and E. coli—pathogens that thrive in animal waste and can find their way into animal-derived food (Hribar 2010, p. 16). Pesticides used on the crops that are then incorporated into animal feed and then into animal flesh are also thought to pose a danger to humans (Goldberg 2016). Animal feeding practices and crowded conditions in factory farms are implicated in illnesses ranging from bacterial infections to various chronic diseases, such as mad cow, and viral infections, such as influenza (Sapkota et al. 2007).

The use of antibiotics in animals destined to become food is especially concerning from a human health standpoint. Most antibiotics sold in the United States, roughly 80 percent, are used in animal agriculture (ConsumersUnion 2016). For the most part, these drugs are not used to fight acute infections in animals, but rather to speed animals' growth and prevent infection. This has led to the development of bacteria that are antibiotic-resistant—the so-called superbugs. In the course of handling raw flesh or eating undercooked meat, these superbugs are sometimes ingested, and this can cause illnesses. These illnesses are exceptionally difficult to cure because the superbugs causing them are resistant to antibiotics. Even if they do not cause illnesses outright, bacteria are uniquely equipped to give their resistance to other bacteria, including those of other genera and species, making it harder to fight a growing number of bacterial diseases (Centers for Disease Control and Prevention 2016).

Additional human health risks stem from the consumption of certain kinds and quantities of animal-derived food, regardless of whether that food began as a cow or pig on a family farm or in a CAFO. The World Health Organization has listed bacon, hot dogs, and sausages as carcinogens (Aubrey 2015). One meta-analysis of health and nutrition research reports: "A strong body of scientific evidence links excess meat consumption, particularly consumption of red and processed meat, with heart disease, stroke, type 2 diabetes, obesity, certain cancers, and earlier death" (John Hopkins Bloomberg School of Public Health 2016, n.p.).

Recent legislation, such as the Healthy, Hunger-Free Kids Act of 2010 (HHFKA), reflects the perceived seriousness of nutrition-related health problems in young people. In the United States in the past 30 years, obesity has more than doubled in children and quadrupled in adolescents, putting more young people at risk for hypertension, heart disease, and diabetes, among other problems (Centers for Disease Control and Prevention 2015). Obesity and its related health risks are closely linked to a high-fat, low-nutrient diet. Animal-based foods are not the only source of dietary fat, nor the only contributor to obesity and obesity-related diseases, but studies show an association between meat eating and obesity and these diseases (Wang and Beydoun 2009). Compared with plant-based food, meat and other animal-derived food are higher in total fat, saturated fat, cholesterol, and total calories, and meat lacks many of the nutritionally key vitamins, minerals, and fiber contained in plant foods (Newby 2009; Sabaté and Wien 2010; Esselstyn 2013). The HHFKA is intended, among other things, to make vegetables and fruits a larger part of students' diets, and it includes numerous provisions, including support for school gardens and farm-to-table programs, to advance that goal. If students eat more plant-based food, the thinking goes, they will gain important nutrients while avoiding unhealthy fats and too many calories.

Often overlooked in discussions about "meat and health" is the health of those who work in animal agriculture. Eye irritation, respiratory illnesses such as bronchitis and asthma, and nausea are caused by exposure to ammonia, which comes from farm animals' waste, as does hydrogen sulfide, a gas that causes throat irritation and, at high exposures, seizures and comas (Kirby 2010). Particulates, such as manure dust, often contain toxins and bacteria and antibiotic-resistant pathogens that cause lung irritation and carry various diseases (ConsumersUnion 2016). Over a quarter of CAFO workers have occupational lung diseases (Gurian-Sherman 2008, p. 60).

Overall, jobs in meat and poultry industries are thought to be among the most dangerous in the United States, and of these, work in slaughterhouses is considered to be especially dangerous (Oxfam 2015). A glimpse into the most common kind of slaughterhouse work indicates why:

The chain is the heartbeat of any meat processing plant, the mechanized driver of eviscerated hogs, cattle and chickens, hung up on hooks and quickly moving down a line at these massive meat factories. Workers disassemble the animals into the cuts consumers prefer – tenderloins and chicken tenders, beef chuck and pork chops.

The workers. . .slaughter and process hundreds of animals an hour, forced to work at high speeds in cold conditions, doing thousands of the same repetitions over and over, with few breaks. That production literally feeds the average American, who eats about 200 pounds of meat a year.

That furious pace also fuels an array of assaults to workers' muscles, tendons, ligaments and nerves called musculoskeletal disorders, or MSDs, causing sprains, strains, pains, or inflammation. (Lowe 2016, n.p.)

## INTERVAL

At some level, by a certain age we all know that eating meat entails the killing of animals. What many may not know, or know only in the most partial and shadowy way, is that meat eating in modern society almost always entails harm to the environment and climate, the suffering of animals prior to slaughter, and risks to the health of humans. It may be assumed that all these problems can be avoided and that it is possible to bypass the CAFO system and eat only organic meat from animals raised humanely on environmentally sustainable farms operated by workers' whose health and safety are carefully protected. In fact, over the past 70 years, CAFOs have come to dominate meat production (Hauter 2012; Conkin 2008). Thus, the average student (along with everyone else who eats meat and other products derived from animals) will almost certainly be eating the flesh of creatures whose lives were spent in CAFOs and ended in slaughterhouses. Through his or her diet, this individual will be contributing to pollution and climate change, animal suffering, and risks to human health, his or her own, and that of others. For most, this contribution is made unconsciously, unknowingly. An integrated outlook on meat consumption is one in which connections encompassing food are brought into focus. Education, a topic to which we now turn, is the most widely recognized process by which such focus is achieved.

## EDUCATIONAL CONSIDERATIONS AND POSSIBILITIES

Most students, in the elementary grades through high school, now have opportunities to learn *something* about food, pollution and climate change, other-than-human animal life, and health risks related to diet. From the perspective of promoting an integrated outlook, however, efforts are needed to help students gain insight into relations between (and within) these elements. If these efforts are fruitful, a student who is beginning to develop an integrated outlook will be better able to consider how various foods bear on different dimensions of the environment, on animal life, and on human health. The student will more frequently see food items not discretely, but in terms of connections and relations. He or she may wonder why and how certain foods have become associated with particular groups or why the school lunch menu regularly includes some items but not others. Or perhaps he or she will inquire into the relation between swelling landfills and school lunch food packaging, examining landfill-bound waste from his or her own school. Perhaps the student will ask about the relation between the edibility of a particular kind of animal flesh and its food status: Why is chicken a food but cat a pet? (Herzog 2010). These are just a few of the possible manifestations of students' integrated outlooks.

Schools might endeavor to help students cultivate a more integrated outlook in a number of ways. Such endeavors, like all other educational endeavors, should take local circumstances into account. But in most cases, even existing resources, particularly the academic disciplines, might be organized in ways that support the cultivation of an integrated outlook among students (Phenix 1964, pp. 311–321). Specifically, the academic disciplines, now usually taught discretely, might be purposely drawn together in ways that maintain the disciplines' integrity while illuminating connections between what initially may seem to be discrete phenomena. In the case of complex phenomena, such as those discussed here, advancing students' insight and understanding will likely require the contributions of several disciplines. For instance, biology and chemistry together could help illuminate the relation between animal waste and acid rain better than either discipline alone. The widespread use of corn in animal feed is made clearer in light of botany and history together; botany illuminates attributes of corn as a plant while history gives insight into the development of agricultural policies supporting corn production over other alternatives. Similarly, nutrition science and anthropology together can help students understand which potential edibles are viewed *as food* for themselves and for others: nutrition science can help students understand the various nutritional qualities of different plants and animals while anthropology sheds light on how different food cultures have developed in different times and places.

The sciences and social sciences have obvious roles in helping students gain an integrated outlook, particularly in respect to the topic at hand, but other school subjects can contribute significantly as well. The arts (including literary arts) are seen as helping to cultivate powers of imagination, broadening moral and intellectual horizons, and fostering sympathy (Moe 2016). Arts stir and awaken. The development of care and concern for the environment, for animals used for food, or for human health will not necessarily follow from encounters with arts, but such encounters provide fertile ground for cultivating these other-oriented attachments. Artistic engagement is not compatible with routine ways of thinking and feeling—or with not thinking or feeling at all.

Then, of course, aspects of the sciences and arts might also be paired, inviting students to consider, say, the scientific and technological aspects of the CAFO and slaughterhouse in terms of human and other-than-human animal experiences. To pick one example, the book *Kira-Kira* (Kadohata 2005), accessible to older children and young adults, includes a depiction of line work in a chicken processing plant. Readers who care about the book's characters will likely find themselves reflecting on the physical and emotional strains entailed in this work—and about those who do this work in the real world. The minds of some readers will no doubt turn toward the birds being "disassembled" at such a furious pace. The cultivation of affective/moral powers such as imagination and sympathy is often reciprocally connected with the cultivation of academic knowledge: sympathy, care, and concern for another may spur the acquisition of knowledge about the other's circumstances and vice versa. It is often difficult to distinguish moral knowledge from academic knowledge because the two are so entwined.

How any content might best be conceptualized, organized, and delivered will depend on the particular features of each educational situation, including teachers' and students' interests, available resources, and broader educational goals. Conventional "teacher and text" centered instruction, hands-on work in science labs, school gardens, and the school cafeteria, field trips, and projects of various kinds are all possibilities; virtual reality experiences, particularly those in which students can assume the vantage point of a cow or pig in a CAFO (e.g., *iAnimal*) may be especially instructive for older students. In recent years, scholars working within eco-justice, critical animal studies, and eco-feminist theoretical frameworks have examined various aspects of the environment and human and other-than-human animal lives in explicitly educational terms, and a number of these scholars have offered analyses of and recommendations for teaching practices that span traditional subject and disciplinary boundaries (Fassbinder et al. 2012; Martusewicz et al. 2015; Rice and Rud 2016). There are also dozens of documentaries, hundreds of popular books, television and radio news stories, tens of thousands of scientific and other academic papers, and countless Internet sources illuminating these connections that teachers might use for instructional purposes.

Developing a more integrated outlook in respect to meat eating requires coming to grips with content that some students—perhaps many students—will find threatening to at least some degree. Because the majority of students are omnivorous, there are many potentially threatening topics related to diet, but most threatening of all are those topics implicating a student's *own* diet in animals' suffering, harms to the environment, and health risks to self and others. No one welcomes the knowledge that their once taken-for-granted noontime hamburger is implicated in cows' misery or industrial workers' exposure to pathogens. Care must be taken to prevent students from rejecting threatening content outright.

Recent research suggests that prefacing instruction that will include potentially threatening content with activities that bolster students' feelings of self-worth may reduce the perception of threat to an extent that students are better able to engage with the content (Graves 2015; Nyhan and Reifler 2016). For example, a teacher might first involve students in non-threatening, pro-animal, pro-environment, or pro-human health activities, perhaps collecting towels or bedding for an animal shelter, planting trees in a new housing development, or conducting a "healthy-eats" food drive. In the context of such activities, students are encouraged to see themselves in a positive light vis-à-vis other animals, the environment, and human health. Thus bolstered, students may be open to considering aspects of their dietary conduct that can be seen as potentially problematic for others or self.

In addition to buttressing students' sense of self-worth prior to discussing potentially threatening content, teachers might introduce this content in a way that does not directly implicate students. For example, teachers might ask students to conduct an investigation into an especially popular animal-based food and inquire into the environmental impact of its manufacture, the conditions under which the animals that become the food are raised and slaughtered, its nutritional value, how the food is packaged, advertised, sold, and so on. A similar investigation might involve the different offerings in the school cafeteria. Or, perhaps, students might be asked to evaluate the interests served by particular food policies, practices, or products or to analyze animals-as-food slogans (e.g., Pork: The other white meat; Beef: It's what for dinner; Tuna: Chicken of the sea) with an eye toward understanding the means by which these slogans work to shape perceptions. Such exercises provide students a window into the industrialized food system and its adjuncts, but they also provide an indirect route by which students may come to see how their own dietary practices fit into this system. Students' own inquiries, especially when guided by insightful and sympathetic teachers, will typically help students perceive more and more connections involving meat-based foods.

Food journal writing provides yet another way to help students address potentially threatening aspects of their own diet. Journal writing is a private activity, where thoughts and feelings can be examined without fear of others' negative judgments. Keeping a journal may help focus students' attention on the emotional and moral dimensions of the food they consume. Writing about experiences, including experiences with food, brings to mind aspects of those experiences that would otherwise likely be taken for granted. It requires the writer to stop and think, rather than to proceed as if on autopilot. Of course, food choices are never made entirely freely; what students choose to eat will almost always be connected in some way to culture and politics and many other factors. While journal writing is a solitary activity, it also enables students to develop thoughts to the point where they might be more confidently shared with others in conversation; it is in such conversation that students are likely to see how their own food experience is shaped by factors that are beyond their immediate, personal control, including food culture, politics, and economics. Students' realization that their dietary experiences are shaped by such powerful forces need not induce resignation or feelings of powerlessness. Indeed, the realization is essential if students are going to participate purposefully in shaping the food system in which their own experiences occur.

## CONCLUDING THOUGHT

We cannot know definitively how students will respond to efforts to help them gain a more integrated outlook on meat, and we cannot know exactly where that experience will lead in the long run. As a result of their educational experiences, perhaps some students will try to change lunch offerings at their own school. Perhaps some will develop an interest in environmentally friendlier approaches to agriculture or pose new ethical challenges to dominant ideas about the relative value of human and other-than-human animal lives. Some students may become lobbyists for industrial agriculture. The outcome of efforts to educate students about diet and the various relations it entails cannot be known with certainty in advance, but the almost certain outcome of failing to try is that students' outlook on one of life's essential activities will remain fragmented.

## NOTE

1. Even if painless, stress-free slaughter is possible, meat eating entails the taking of animal life, which itself raises profound ethical questions. These questions are beyond the scope of this essay.

## REFERENCES

Aubrey, A. (2015, October 26). Bad day for bacon: Processed meats cause cancer, WHO Says. *The Salt*. Retrieved from http://www.npr.org/sections/the-salt/2015/10/26/451211964/bad-day-for-bacon-processed-red-meats-cause-cancer-says-who

Castle, S., & Goodman, A. (2014). *The meaty truth: Why our food is destroying our health and environment—And who is responsible*. New York: Skyhorse.

Centers for Disease Control and Prevention. (2015, August 27). *Childhood obesity facts*. Retrieved from http://www.cdc.gov/healthyschools/obesity/facts.htm

Centers for Disease Control and Prevention. (2016). *Antibiotic use in food-producing animals*. Retrieved from http://www.cdc.gov/narms/animals.html

Clark, B., Stewart, G. B., Panzone, L. A., Kyriazakis, L. A., & Frewer, L. J. (2016). A systematic review of public attitudes, perceptions and behaviours towards production diseases associated with farm animal welfare. *Journal of Agricultural and Environmental Ethics, 29*(3), 455–478. https://doi.org/10.1007/s10806-016-9615-x. Retrieved from http://link.springer.com/article/10.1007/s 10806-016-9615-x.

Coe, S. (1995). *Dead meat*. New York: Four Walls Eight Windows Publishing.

Conkin, P. K. (2008). *A revolution down on the farm: The transformation of American agriculture since 1929*. Lexington: University of Kentucky Press.

ConsumersUnion. (2016). *The overuse of antibiotics in food animals threatens public health*. Retrieved from http://consumersunion.org/news/the-overuse-of-antibiotics-in-food-animals-threatens-public-health-2/

Eisnitz, G. A. (2007). *Slaughterhouse: The shocking story of greed, neglect, and inhumane treatment inside the U.S. meat industry*. New York: Prometheus.

Esselstyn, R. (2013). *My beef with meat: The healthiest argument for eating a plant-strong diet*. New York: Hachette.

Farr, S. (2015). *Beyond the factory farm: How slaughterhouses are polluting the planet*. Retrieved from http://www.onegreenplanet.org/environment/how-slaughterhouses-are-polluting-the-planet/

Faruqi, S. (2015). *Project animal farm: An accidental journey into the secret world of farming and the truth about our food*. New York: Pegasus.

Fassbinder, S., Nocella, A. J., & Kahn, R. (Eds.). (2012). *Greening the academy: Ecopedagogy through the liberal arts*. Rotterdam: The Netherlands: Sense Publishers.

Foer, J. S. (2009). *Eating animals*. New York: Little Brown.

Food Empowerment Project. (2016). *Pollution (Water, Air, Chemicals)*. Retrieved from http://www.foodispower.org/pollution-water-air-chemicals/

Genoways, T. (2014). *The chain: Farm, factory, and the fate of our food*. New York: HarperCollins.

Global Change Research Program. (2014). *2014 National climate assessment*. Washington, DC: Global Change Research Program. Retrieved from http://nca2014.globalchange.gov/report/our-changing-climate/introduction#intro-section

Goldberg, A. G. (2016). Farm animal welfare and human health. *Current Environmental Health, 3*(3), 313–321. Retrieved from http://link.springer.com/article/10.1007/s40572-016-0097-9.

Graves, C. (2015, February 20). Why debunking myths about vaccines hasn't convinced dubious parents. *Harvard Business Review*. Retrieved from https://hbr.org/2015/02/why-debunking-myths-about-vaccines-hasnt-convinced-dubious-parents

Gurian-Sherman, D. (2008). *CAFOs uncovered: The untold costs of animal feeding operations* Cambridge: Union of Concerned Scientists. Retrieved from http://www.ucsusa.org/sites/default/files/legacy/assets/documents/food_and_agriculture/cafos-uncovered.pdf

Hauter, W. (2012). *Foodopoly: The battle over the future of food and farming in America*. New York: The New Press.

Herzog, H. (2010). *Some we love, some we hate, some we eat*. New York: HarperCollins.

Hribar, C. (2010). *Understanding concentrated animal feeding operations and their impact on communities* (pp. 2–5). Bowling Green: National Association of Local Boards of Health. Retrieved from https://www.cdc.gov/nceh/ehs/docs/understanding_cafos_nalboh.pdf

Humane Society of the United States. (2015, June 25). *Farm animal statistics: Slaughter totals*. Retrieved from http://www.humanesociety.org/news/resources/research/stats_slaughter_totals.html

Imhoff, D. (Ed.). (2010). *The CAFO reader: The tragedy of industrial animal factories*. Berkeley: University of California Press.

John Hopkins Bloomberg School of Public Health. (2016). *Health and environmental implications of U.S. meat consumption and production*. Baltimore: John Hopkins University. Retrieved from https://www.jhsph.edu/research/centers-and-institutes/johns-hopkins-center-for-a-livable-future/projects/meatless_monday/resources/meat_consumption.html

Kadohata, C. (2005). *Kira-Kira*. New York: Atheneum Books.
Kirby, D. (2010). *Animal factory: The looming threat of industrial pig, dairy, and poultry farms to humans and the environment*. New York: St. Martin's Press.
Leonard, C. (2014). *The meat racket: The secret takeover of America's food business*. New York: NY. Simon & Schuster.
Lowe, P. (2016, July 14). Working 'the chain,' slaughterhouse workers face life-long injuries. *Harvest Public Media*. Retrieved from http://harvestpublicmedia.org/article/working-chain-slaughterhouse-workers-face-life-long-injuries
Lymbery, P. (2014). *Farmageddon: The true cost of cheap meat*. London: Bloomsbury.
Martusewicz, R. A., Edmundson, J., & Lupinacci, J. (Eds.). (2015). *EcoJustice education: Toward diverse, democratic, and sustainable communities* (2nd ed.). New York: Routledge.
Moe, A. M. (2016). The work of literature in a multispecies world. In S. Rice & A. G. Rud (Eds.), *The educational significance of human and non-human animal interactions* (pp. 133–149). New York: Palgrave.
Newby, P. K. (2009). Plant food and plant-based diets: Protective against childhood obesity? *American Journal of Clinical Nutrition, 89*(5), 1572S–1587S.
Nyhan, B., & Reifler, J. (2016, September 15). *The roles of information deficits and identity threat in the prevalence of misperceptions*. Retrieved from http://www.dartmouth.edu/~nyhan/opening-political-mind.pdf
Oxfam. (2015). *Lives on the line: The human cost of cheap chicken*. Boston: Oxfam America. Retrieved from https://www.oxfamamerica.org/static/media/files/Lives_on_the_Line_Full_Report_Final.pdf
Pachirat, T. (2011). *Every twelve seconds: Industrialized slaughter and the politics of sight*. New Haven: Yale University Press.
Pew Commission. (2016, August 3). *Environmental impact of industrial farm animal production*. Pew Commission on Industrial Farm Animal Production Fansite. Retrieved from http://www.ncifap.org/_images/212-4_EnvImpact_tc_Final.pdf
Phenix, P. H. (1964). *Realms of meaning: A philosophy of the curriculum for general education*. New York: McGraw-Hill.
Pitney, N. (2016, October 28). Scientists believe the chickens we eat are being slaughtered while conscious. *The Huffington Post*. Retrieved from http://www.huffingtonpost.com/entry/chickens-slaughtered-conscious_us_580e3d35e4b000d0b157bf98
Rice, S., & Rud, A. G. (Eds.). (2016). *The educational significance of human and non-human animal interactions: Blurring the species line*. New York: Palgrave Macmillan.
Sabaté, J., & Wien, M. (2010, March 17). Vegetarian diets and childhood obesity prevention. *American Journal of Clinical Nutrition, 91*(5), 1525S–1529S. Retrieved from http://ajcn.nutrition.org/content/91/5/1525S

Sapkota, A. R., Lefferts, L. Y., McKenzie, S., & Walker, P. (2007). What do we feed to food-production animals? A review of animal feed ingredients and their potential impacts on human health. *Environmental Health Perspectives, 115*(5): 663–670. Published online 2007 Feb 8. doi: https://doi.org/10.1289/ehp.9760., http://www.ncbi.nlm.nih.gov/pmc/articles/PMC1867957/

Solotaroff, P. (2013, December 10). The belly of the beast: The dirty truth about cheap meat. *RollingStone*. Retrieved from http://www.rollingstone.com/feature/belly-beast-meat-factory-farms-animal-activists

Stahler, C. (2010). *How many youth are vegetarian? The vegetarian resource group asks in a 2010 National Poll*. Baltimore: Vegetarian Resource Group. Retrieved from http://www.vrg.org/press/youth_poll_2010.php

Tietz, J. (2006, December 14). Boss hog: The dark side of America's top pork producer. *RollingStone*. Retrieved from http://www.rollingstone.com/culture/news/boss-hog-the-dark-side-of-americas-top-pork-producer-20061214

U.S. Government Accountability Office. (2016). *Workplace safety and health: Additional data needed to address continued hazards in the meat and poultry industry*. Washington, DC: U.S. Government. Retrieved from http://www.gao.gov/assets/680/676796.pdf.

United Nations Food and Agriculture Organization. (2006). *Livestock's long shadow: Environmental issues and options*. Retrieved from http://www.fao.org/docrep/010/a0701e/a0701e00.htm

Wang, Y., & Beydoun, M. A. (2009). Meat consumption is associated with obesity and central obesity among US adults. *International Journal of Obesity, 33*, 621–628. doi:10.1038/ijo.2009.45; published online 24 March 2009.

# CHAPTER 8

# "Social Consequences" of School Lunch for Students Who Receive Special Education Services: A Critical Outlook

*Susan M. Bashinski and Kipton D. Smilie*

A curious absence exists in Susan Levine's (2008) *School Lunch Politics: The Surprising History of America's Favorite Welfare Program*. In her comprehensive account of school lunch programs in the United States, Levine places particular attention on federal legislation, including laws enacted in the early decades of the twentieth century to regulations in place today. All in all, Levine examines nine pieces of federal legislation, but one federal mandate, the *Individuals with Disabilities Education Act* (IDEA) (2004), receives no mention from Levine. In fact, Levine provides no discussion of students who receive special education services and their experiences in the lunchroom. This absence is particularly notable as Levine's history of the school lunch program is marked by specific student populations and their influence by, and reaction to, policy and regulations. Levine examines the school lunch program's aim to feed children from poorer households. She details early attempts to Americanize immigrant students by providing "American" fare, and she chronicles the challenges and roadblocks immigrant students encountered as they tried to participate in the school lunch program. As Levine (2008) writes, the school lunch program

S. M. Bashinski (✉) • K. D. Smilie
Missouri Western State University, St. Joseph, MO, USA

© The Author(s) 2018
S. Rice, A. G. Rud (eds.), *Educational Dimensions of School Lunch*,
https://doi.org/10.1007/978-3-319-72517-8_8

135

is inextricably connected with many "at-risk" student populations. Yet, students who receive special education (SPED) services are not included in this particular historical review.

## STUDENT POPULATIONS IN THE LUNCHROOM: INTERACTIONS AND EXCHANGES

Generally missing in school lunch literature are studies of the lunchroom social experiences of students who receive special education services. In the past two decades, scholars have begun focusing on the social interactions and status dynamics at play during lunch involving students' gender, age, race, social class, and culture. Barrie Thorne (1993), in *Gender Play: Girls and Boys in School*, examines the roles and meanings of gender and age with elementary students. While "parents, teachers, and other adults" play a major role in the socialization of children, Thorne argues that "children's collective activities should weigh more fully in our overall understanding of gender and social life" (p. 4). She pays particular attention to the playground and cafeteria because these spaces allow students to form their own groups (in contrast to classrooms where teachers often form groups based on students' perceived abilities). Thorne argues that we can learn much from observations on the playground and in the lunchroom precisely because of the freedom these contexts provide. Thorne notes that "eating together is a prime emblem of solidarity, and each day at lunchtime there is a fresh scramble as kids deliberately choose where, and with whom, to eat" (p. 42). Such choice reveals much about the social interconnectedness among students. Thorne contends that "social hierarchies have a loose relationship to somatic type" (p. 140); in lunchrooms, students are ultimately "freer to shape the grounds of interaction" (p. 161).

Penelope Eckert (1989) reports her ethnographic study of high schools and their lunchrooms in *Jocks and Burnouts: Social Categories and Identity in the High School*. Like Thorne (1993), Eckert (1989) considers the lunchroom as a space encompassing various social meanings and values. Eckert pays close attention to two perennial cliques in high schools: the "jocks" and the "burnouts." In her study, Eckert finds that the jocks and the burnouts comprise a relatively small number of students, but that these two cliques possess social power and influence that reverberate throughout most of the student population. The jocks typically come from higher socio-economic status (SES) backgrounds, make better grades, participate in more school activities and events, and attend college at a higher rate. The burnouts, on the other hand, come from lower SES backgrounds, typically receive lower grades, take more vocational courses, and generally reject school activities and events. The jocks "center their social lives in the school and accept the school as a 'home away from home,'" (p. 51), while the burnouts' marginalized position is illustrated through "their rejection of the school as a comprehensive social institution" (p. 51). The lunchroom, Eckert illustrates, is a space where jocks and burnouts enact their respective identities. The jocks use the lunchroom to eat and to interact with fellow jocks, while the burnouts generally try to eschew the lunchroom in order to "express their counter-cultural position in the school" (p. 51) in favor of congregating in off-limit spaces, such as the parking lot and vocational classrooms. Ultimately, according to Eckert, the burnouts seek to "reject school facilities that represent the school's in loco parentis role" (p. 51). The burnouts deplore the quality of food served in the lunchroom, though the jocks generally find the food acceptable. Eckert sees this as the burnouts' rejection of "the school's parental role of providing food and living space, namely, lockers and the cafeteria" (p. 51).

Eckert (1989) characterizes the lunchroom in one additional respect: as a place of social networking. In her study, Eckert witnesses the imposition of seating arrangements in classrooms. As Thorne (1993) notes, the lunchroom provides one space in which social networks can flourish in an unfettered fashion. But, as Eckert (1989) explains, such freedom brings social dangers. When Eckert examines students with "limited networks" (i.e., those students with few friends and low status), she finds that "lunchtime can be a difficult and painful time" (p. 46). This sentiment is echoed in the work of Heyne et al. (2012), who write, "lunchtime can be a source of anxiety for students with disabilities, as it can be for any student" (p. 56). Social interactions between students who experience disabilities and those who do not are not likely to occur without structured support. Those students with a small social circle face a lunchroom with few personal connections. For Eckert (1989), such a student

> who eats alone or walks in the halls alone during this period of heightened visibility is stigmatized. Those who find themselves alone manage as best they can by making themselves inconspicuous, drifting as an unwelcome guest among established groups, or simply hiding. They do not, however, escape notice. (p. 46)

Donna Eder (1995) also explores social networks in the lunchroom in *School Talk: Gender and Adolescent Culture*. The lunchroom, for Eder and her research team, "bears the clear mark of adolescent peer culture" (p. 19) as a space that "represents student, not adult, territory" (p. 20). Voluntary seating arrangements and "saving seats" both define and enforce group behavior. As a result, Eder and her research team note "because seating arrangements were continually negotiated, we saw open attempts to include and exclude certain students" (p. 24). Students who received special education services often were in an isolated group since "they were placed in separate classrooms at the time of the study, which made it difficult for them to form other friendships" (p. 26). This is one such way in which classroom associations, or lack thereof, influence lunchroom dynamics since many students who receive special education services sit by themselves, leading Eder and her research team to deem these students "isolates." In describing "isolates," Eder and her team note that this group exhibits characteristics that are perceived negatively and "made special education students more likely candidates for social isolation" (p. 49). Eder's research team details an incident in which a student with a disability, sitting by herself, is approached by groups of two to five students during a 15-minute period. The lone student is told that other students "liked" her, and one boy repeatedly asks her if she knew "what a homosexual was" (p. 76); some students act as if they are "poisoned" by being close to her. Such an onslaught creates much laughter among other students in the lunchroom, leaving the student with a disability "really shaken."

Murray Milner (2004) takes a more sociological approach in his ethnographic *Freaks, Geeks, and Cool Kids: American Teenagers, Schools, and the Culture of Consumption*. Milner and his research team studied a large high school over the course of two years. Through this study, Milner develops his theory of status relations, which helps to articulate *"why status groups have the particular characteristics that make them different from other types of stratified groups"* and *"why a relationship between two people or two groups may focus on status differences in one situation but ignore them in another"* (p. 182). Like Eckert's 1989 study of the jocks and burnouts, Milner's (2004) study of social cliques finds particular relevance in the freedom of the lunchroom. Initially Milner notes that, in general, those who are most vulnerable are harassed the most, and he expresses particular concern over the treatment of students who receive special education services, saying that "one of the most troubling things is the aggressive harassment of the physically or mentally handicapped [*sic*]" (p. 89). As Eder (1995) explains, students who receive special education services may not be involved with peers from general education, even during class times. The lunchroom provides a setting for the participation of the marginalized, perceived "weak students," allowing those in a social group seeking increased status to show off their power in public. Milner (2004) posits a few reasons as to why the most demeaning behavior is directed toward the weakest and most defenseless. Hostility is often exhibited "by scapegoating the vulnerable...and the vulnerable offer an opportunity to hone and display one's skills without risking significant retaliation" (p. 90). Most disturbing, though, is Milner's theory that because the high school social scene places such an enormous value on conformity, then "deviance must be persecuted lest it call into question the basic assumptions of the normative structure. Many handicapped learners [*sic*] do deviate considerably from the norms of other learners. Apparently, this is seen as highly threatening and is punished" (p. 90).

Milner (2004) additionally notes "a tendency for the weakest members of the group to be the most isolated" (p. 90) (similar to the arguments presented by Eder and colleagues in 1995). Milner argues, however, that this exclusion is not always a form of persecution. His observations point to students who receive special education services, who "often do deviate in ways that are at best insensitive to others" (p. 91). Infrequent exposure to students who receive special education services can cause students who receive only general education services to feel uncomfortable, particularly in the openness of the lunchroom. Milner warns, however, that

> reducing the exclusion and isolation of the lowest strata – even handicapped learners [*sic*] in schools – is rarely simply a matter of reducing inequality and changing the prejudices of higher status strata. This is, however, a crucial prerequisite to greater inclusion and solidarity. (p. 92)

Milner places much focus on the space of the lunchroom, as this space is often contested between various social groups. Fights in the lunchroom occur because "chairs and tables are often scarce" (p. 106). He details that "students confront one another about being in 'their place'" (p. 106), but space is also negotiated through walking and "stalking out territory" (p. 107) during lunch time.

Essentially, walking consists of individuals or groups circulating among more stationary groups of individuals. Some form of this is common in many societies. Territoriality is the claiming of space as a group's own, and the ability to enforce this spatial differentiation. Both are, in part, strategies to control visibility. Visibility is a prerequisite to a distinctive status – high or low. (p. 107)

Milner further illustrates that students eat as quickly as possible in order to create more time for "walking from group to group visiting, gossiping, and flirting" (p. 107). Milner explains that students with high status utilize walking in the lunchroom

because it enables them to maximize their visibility among many groups and individuals who are all part of a contiguous social network. Since they are high status and recognized by many people, moving about helps to maximize their visibility and contacts. (p. 107)

For students with low status, walking serves a similar function. Instead of walking to be seen by all, students with low status walk in order to "attract the attention" (p. 107) of particular higher status groups. He notes that this often occurs for romantic purposes, as students with lower status hope to "bump into" students of a higher status. In "stalking out territory" (p. 107), status groups "focus on defining boundaries, membership, norms, and styles of their group" (p. 108). Milner remarks on the "loyalty to this space" (p. 108) formulated by status groups. Instead of walking, these status groups choose to "mark their territory" (p. 108) with backpacks, notebooks, and even painting their lunchroom tables. Milner summarizes that the "key theoretical point is that in a pluralistic setting, the relevant status arenas may vary for different groups as well as the modes of acquiring status. Where groups use the same arenas and mechanisms, conflict and hostility are more likely" (p. 108).

Beverly Daniel Tatum (1997) explores territory and identity in *Why Are All the Black Kids Sitting Together in the Cafeteria? And Other Conversations about Race*. Tatum examines why "in racially mixed schools all over the country, Black kids were still sitting together in school cafeterias" (p. xvii). She contends that in elementary schools, we can observe "young children of diverse racial backgrounds playing with one another, sitting at the snack table together, crossing racial boundaries with an ease uncommon in adolescence" (p. 52). She investigates this "clustering by race" throughout her work, particularly its manifestation in the lunch-room in middle schools and high schools. Tatum notes that a lunchroom table including only Black students, who are "collectively embodying an oppositional stance" (p. 62), causes many administrators to question "why they are sitting together [and] what can be done to prevent it" (p. 62). Tatum argues that such a clustering by Black students at a lunchroom table serves as a type of force or strength in the overall school structure, especially if Black students constitute a minority of the student population. This self-segregation by older students, as also noted by Milner (2004), constitutes a means of solidarity. Tatum (1997) witnesses the same phenomenon in the corporate world, as "even mature adults sometimes need to connect with someone who looks like them and who shares the same experiences" (p. 88). This structuring shows that "within-group dialogue can often be as important, and sometimes more important, than between-group dialogue" (p. 218). Adolescent students, though, often struggle with their identities and the meanings attached to them; Tatum cites "the constructive potential that informed adults can have in the identity development process" (p. 69). She goes on to provide an example of how a teacher realized a student's "need for a same-race peer group and helped her find one" (p. 69).

## MARGINALIZATION OF STUDENTS WHO EXPERIENCE DISABILITY THROUGHOUT HISTORY

Though several scholars have investigated the interactions and vulnerabilities of various social and "at risk" groups in the school lunchroom, their work has not considered the influence of disability (Eckert 1989; Levine 2008; Tatum 1997; Thorne 1993; Weaver-Hightower 2011). In fact, very little research considers the ways in which students who receive special education services function within the freer space of the lunchroom environment. As Milner (2004) notes, the most likely targets of bullies are those students who are viewed as "most vulnerable." It seems ironic that students who experience disabilities, by very definition a potentially vulnerable group at increased risk of social marginalization, has been examined in research to only a minimal degree (e.g., Eder 1995).

Before we specifically discuss the participation of students who receive special education services in public school lunch programs in the present day, a brief review of the historical view and treatment of individuals who experience disabilities, particularly physical or intellectual disabilities, is in order. The earliest identified work addressing issues—*any* issues—associated with disability is attributed to Aristotle (cited in Furlow 1973): "As to the exposure and rearing of children, let there be a law that no deformed child shall live." Sadly, this quotation reflects the pervasive historical perspective that individuals who experience physical or intellectual disabilities are "lesser" beings in one way or another. In many societies throughout history, individuals who experience disability have not been treated as "human." These persons have been abandoned to die, forced into service, drowned/burned during the period of the Inquisition (Kunc and Van der Klift 1995), and gassed during the Nazi regime (estimated at 80,000+) (Smith and Wehmeyer 2012).

In the United States in the early 1900s, attitudes toward individuals who experienced disability were clearly negative. The infamous Kallikak study (published in 1912 regarding a family in rural New Jersey) linked mental retardation,[1] heredity, and criminality (Smith and Wehmeyer 2012). Remnants of this line of thinking persist to this day, sometimes resulting in the wrongful incarceration of individuals with disability, particularly intellectual disability (ID) (Perske 1991), or young adults with challenging behaviors. Cases of persons with ID wrongfully confessing to crimes they could not have committed are not uncommon, possibly because these individuals lacked understanding, felt too apologetic, or tried too hard to please the police.

Individuals with disability, particularly ID, have been victimized by "politically charged rhetoric and policies, resulting in…institutionalization and forced sterilization" (Smith and Wehmeyer 2012, p. xii). Segregation, frequently in the form of institutionalization, was, historically, often the proposed solution for separating those with physical or intellectual disabilities from the general population (Smith 1995, p. ix). Public schools in the United States often reflect American society. Similar to the movement to provide separate residential facilities (i.e., housing) for persons who experience disabilities, the late nineteenth century saw segregated educational programs emerge for these individuals. The first separate class created solely for students who experienced disabilities is *believed* to have opened in Cleveland, sometime during the period 1874–1879; consensus agreement confirms that a class was established for students with physical or intellectual disabilities in Providence, Rhode Island, in 1896 (Kanner 1964). In many instances, separate classes evolved into segregated educational facilities. (A number of segregated schools, and even more segregated special education classrooms, continue to exist to the present day.) An interesting finding of the President's Committee on Mental Retardation (1970) suggested the idea of the "six-hour retarded child"—that is, a student was *only* viewed as "deficient" or "defective" during the time he or she spent in a special education classroom at school.

The first formalized step toward creating a meaningful place for students who experience disability, of any degree or any type, in the nation's public schools was taken by the United States Congress in 1975 with the passage of the original federal special education (SPED) law (Gargiulo and Bouck 2018; Hallahan et al. 2015; Turnbull et al. 2016). This landmark legislation provided the first mandate for free, appropriate, public education for students with disabilities. Through subsequent reauthorizations and amendments, this law (now known as the Individuals with Disabilities Education Improvement Act of 2004 [IDEA]) provides services for students who experience disabilities, from birth through 21 years of age.

Though segregated schools have been closed or reduced in number, since the passage and reauthorizations of IDEA (1975 through 2004), these persist in several states. The maintenance of segregated special education classrooms/programs is even more pervasive. Although the stated purpose of segregated classrooms was

> to help students with disabilities learn skills and appropriate behavior, the very act of removing students with disabilities from the other students necessarily teaches them that "they are not good enough to belong as they are" and that the privilege of belonging will be granted back to them once they have acquired an undefined number of skills. (Kunc 1992, p. 5)

Though history documents human beings' tendency to segregate persons thought to be sufficiently different from themselves is a common response (Smith 1995), this particular delivery model of special education services seems to reinforce the notion that students must "earn the right to belong" in situations with general education peers—a premise in total contradiction to Maslow's (1970) widely accepted hierarchy in humanistic psychology, which describes "belonging" as a basic human need for love and acceptance. Kunc (1992) views "belonging" as not only an essential human need, but as "a basic human right" (p. 5)—not something which must be earned. Kunc further states that earning the right to belong is not limited to schools, but rather, an expectation that permeates American society—and it is important to remember that practices in US public schools reflect

American society. It seems reasonable to raise the question regarding whether the provision of professional, specialized services might, sometimes, result in "disabling help" (McKnight 1995, p. 36).

The 2004 authorization of IDEA took a significant step toward meaningful "inclusion" of students who experience disabilities in general education programs, by reversing the previous requirement that educational teams justify the amount of time a student who received special education services *spent with* general education peers. With the current iteration of the federal law (IDEA 2004), teams must now justify any amount of time a student who receives special education services in a setting that is *removed from* general education peers (Gargiulo and Bouck 2018; Turnbull et al. 2016). This justification is legally required to be all-encompassing—that is, to address not only time away from peers who are typically developing in core academic and elective classes, but also relative to school bus transportation, extra-curricular activities, the playground, and school lunch.

The placement settings of choice under IDEA (2004) are clearly inclusion in general education environments, with students who have disabilities participating "alongside their nondisabled peers in academic, extracurricular, and (all) other school activities….to the maximum extent appropriate" (Turnbull et al. 2016). The latest trend in meeting the requirements of IDEA (2004) has been described as "full inclusion," which involves all students, who experience all types and degrees of disability, receiving necessary support and remaining in general education settings at their neighborhood schools 100% of the time. This stance is controversial in the field of special education (Gargiulo and Bouck 2018). Arguing for or against full inclusion is beyond the scope of this chapter. Nonetheless it can be agreed that, under current special education law, all students who experience disability are to receive as normalized an educational experience as possible and appropriate. Arbitrary segregationist practices, or policies enacted out of habit, are inequitable for students with a disability. "A central tenet of inclusive education is that belonging is an inherent need of all people and must not be reserved solely for the 'best of us'" (Kunc 1995, p. 10). He goes on to state that including students who experience disability, without valuing their diversity, is an inappropriate application of Maslow's hierarchy in support of inclusive education. Kunc (1992, 1995) appeals to schools to see disability as simply another variable of diversity—not a deficit.

## SOCIAL CONSEQUENCES OF SCHOOL LUNCH—A CALL FOR ACTION

Critical considerations of the lunchroom as a social space to be navigated and negotiated exist in limited number. Marcus B. Weaver-Hightower (2011) essentially issued a "call to action" when he called for more research regarding the social implications of food in schools, writing "although food is ever present, its role in the life of schools has been little studied by education scholars" (p. 15). Weaver-Hightower contends that the social component of food is sorely lacking, and argues that food should be considered "an integral component of the ecology of education – the broader interconnectedness of actors, relationships, conditions, and processes of which education is composed" (p. 16). Of particular interest is Bourdieu's 1984 observation that "food establishes who we are in gendered, sexualized, racial, and ethnic senses, and who we are through food has social consequences" (as cited in Weaver-Hightower 2011, p. 18). This is just as true in school cafeterias as it is in the larger society.

In the aforementioned studies, scholars consider the lunchroom as an often-contested social space. Where students sit and with whom carry significant meanings within the social hierarchy of the school. While a limited number of studies addressing the social consequences of school lunch include a consideration of students who receive special education services, none focuses specifically on the navigation of the lunchroom social space relative to this particular student population. Many of the complexities inherent in social components of the lunchroom would seem to be even more significant for students who receive special education services. For this group of students we might ask, most basically: When do they eat? Where do they eat? With whom do they eat? How do they receive their food? How do they pay? Or which policies and procedures seek to influence their school lunch experience?

Beyond these considerations, though, more complex questions (many of which are raised by the aforementioned scholars) need to be asked regarding the population of students who receive special education services. How do these students navigate the "bodily spaces" of the lunchroom? How do they manage the daily "scramble" for seating described by Thorne (1993)? How penetrable or impenetrable are social networks in the lunchroom, particularly for the group of students Eder and colleagues (1995) referred to as "isolates?" Does visibility or invisibility in the lunchroom, as discussed by both Eckert (1989) and Milner (2004), have particular meaning(s) for students who receive special education services? During school lunch times, students are accustomed to eating with familiar people and seeing objects familiar to their home mealtime environments (e.g., plates, forks, spoons, napkins). But would the school lunch experience change in any significant way if students were to be exposed to unfamiliar people or circumstances (e.g., a student who uses a wheelchair, one who is unable to maneuver a fork, a student who eats via a gastrostomy tube)? What kinds of relationships are created, strengthened, and diminished in the school lunchroom time and space between students who receive special education services and their general education peers?

## SOCIAL CONSEQUENCES OF SCHOOL LUNCH AND STUDENTS WHO RECEIVE SPECIAL EDUCATION SERVICES

For reasons discussed earlier in this chapter, primarily the relative lack of investigation into the lunchroom experiences of students who receive special education services (Eckert 1989; Lauer 2014; Levine 2008; Thorne 1993) and the widespread historical marginalization of individuals with disabilities in US society, we believed it was important to examine policies and procedures that shape school lunch practices in the present day.

Our study involved an electronic survey, created in Google Forms, consisting of 17 questions. Fifteen questions, each of which included a list of bulleted choices, required a response from the participant. Eight questions allowed only one answer; seven instructed the respondent to "check all that apply." The last two, optional survey questions, were short answer inquiries. All questions concerned aspects of the school district's policies and practices associated with school lunch—for both students who receive special education services and those who do not.

The Institutional Review Board of our university approved the study, as did the Institutional Review Boards of two participating school districts. The two Midwestern school districts that participated in this investigation are categorized as "large, urban districts" by the National Center for Educational Statistics (2009)—the federal entity mandated by Congress to compile all data pertinent to public education in the United States. Of the 16,330 local school districts in the United States at the time of this report, 850 were considered to be large, urban districts with enrollments of 10,000 or more students (National Center for Educational Statistics 2009). The two participant districts, hereafter referred to as "District A" and "District B," reported enrollments of students who received special education services, during the 2016–2017 school year, as 11.35% of all students (District A) and 13.35% (District B).

A link to the survey was distributed to the two school district Directors of Special Education Services, along with a note from the authors. These directors were asked to email the survey link to all special education teachers and paraprofessionals, all related services personnel (e.g., speech-language pathologists, occupational therapists, etc.), and all building administrators, whose schools housed any sort of special education program. The survey was distributed to 246 and 214 recipients, in Districts A and B, respectively. Approximately two weeks later (i.e., 15 days in District A; 20 days in District B), the survey link was distributed one more time (to all initial recipients, since all responses were anonymous).

A total of 54.8% of surveys distributed were returned (252 responses received/460 sent). Personnel employed by District A returned 42.3% of distributed surveys; District B employees responded at a rate of 69.2%—both very respectable survey return rates. Individuals with nine different areas of training/expertise completed and returned the survey; the largest single group of respondents, as expected, was special education teachers ($n$ = 158). The second largest number of survey responses was received from school administrators ($n$ = 28). See Fig. 8.1 for a breakdown of responses received, by participants' roles in the schools.

It is especially interesting to note that, even though the final two, write-in survey questions were optional, 175 respondents (i.e., 69.4%) provided at least one substantive answer to the question, "What have you observed, if anything, in terms of social consequences of the ways in which learners who receive SPECIAL EDUCATION services participate in the school lunch program?" The final question, "Is there anything else you feel is important regarding school lunch for learners who receive SPECIAL EDUCATION services, which has not been addressed here?" received specific comments from 49 participants (i.e., 19.4%). (Responses such as "none," "nothing," or "n/a" were *not* included in either of the comments counts.) Answers received to this last question led us to conclude that the survey appeared to be comprehensive in its coverage—in fact, one respondent wrote "I think this is (a) complete survey," and another offered thanks for "allowing us to participate in this survey."

Although a detailed analysis of all qualitative comments is neither appropriate nor possible here, it is possible to give a general sense of respondents' perceptions of the lunchroom experiences of students who

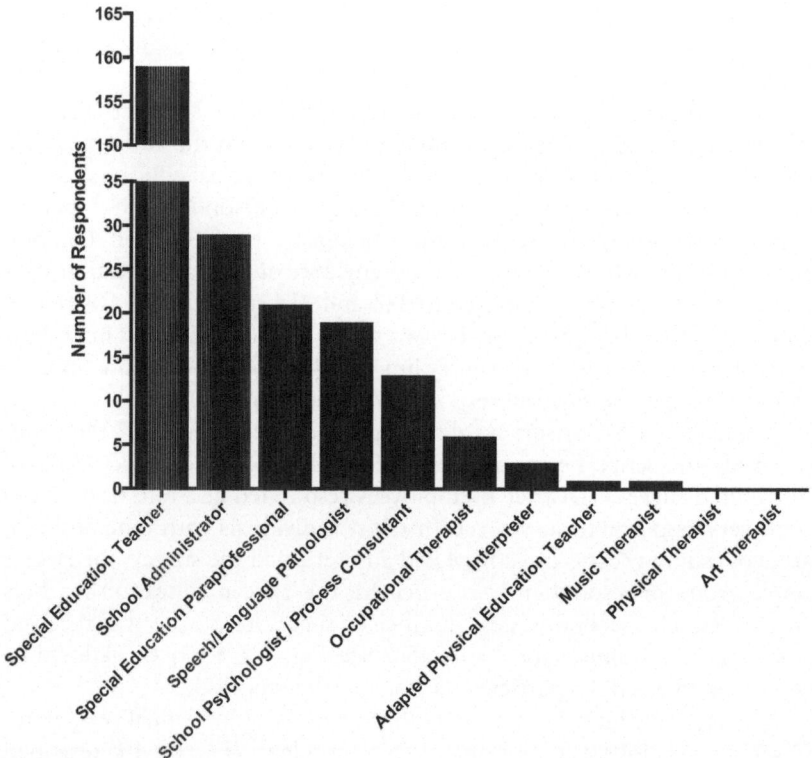

**Fig. 8.1**  Respondent roles

receive special education services. Representative positive comments included, "I haven't seen any child that receives SPED services being objected [*sic*] to negative consequences during lunch due to their [*sic*] disability. It's a table of kids, not over here are the reg ed kids and over there are the sped kids" (pre-K/elementary SPED teacher), "General education students interact with students receiving SPED services which improves social skills for both" (elementary/middle school speech-language pathologist), "All kids need to eat lunch together" (high school SPED teacher).

A few examples of representative negative comments included, "Some students experience social difficulties in the cafeteria with finding a group to sit with and engaging in appropriate conversation during the lunch period" (middle/high school psychologist/consultant), "I have noticed that...students who are placed in a more restrictive environment may not have as many choices or will eat in the classroom. I feel that some of these students do not get the social aspects that they deserve" (elementary school SPED teacher), "I have seen negative social consequences for students that have lunch during their SPED classes. Small groups of special education students are uncomfortable when they go to lunch and are expected to sit at a table meant for 12, when there is [sic] only a few of them.... A group of 6th graders (from a different teacher) didn't want to even go to lunch. They would also return from lunch 5–10 minutes early because they didn't want to sit there, isolated from the rest of the students" (middle school SPED teacher).

In the body of survey responses on the whole, positive comments significantly outnumbered negative comments or concerns quantitatively. In many respects, in this limited sample of two school districts, it would appear that *some* positive social consequences emanate from the school lunch experiences of many students who receive special education services. In addition to the limitation of a relatively small sample size, we question whether some survey respondents might have misinterpreted "social consequences" to mean "behavioral consequences" for manifestation of socially inappropriate behaviors.

Regardless of these two limitations of this school lunch survey, one very significant finding resoundingly emerged in response to the question, "How are school lunch policies/procedures for the majority of learners who receive SPECIAL EDUCATION services determined?" Respondents were allowed to choose only one best answer to this question. In particular, the responses of the 28 school administrators, exactly one-half ($n = 14$) answered that school lunch policy and procedures were "determined by school district policy" (eight from District A [47.1% of administrators who responded] and six from District B [54.5%]). The remaining 14 administrator-respondents provided one of the six other answers (see Fig. 8.2). Anecdotally, 14 of 28 administrators noted that students in general education could "sit anywhere in the cafeteria," but zero answered in this manner in regard to students who receive SPED services; 19 of 28 administrators responded that students who receive SPED services have assigned tables in the school lunchroom.

By contrast, in response to the question, "How are school lunch policies/procedures for the majority of learners who receive SPECIAL EDUCATION services determined?" only 34.3% of non-administrator

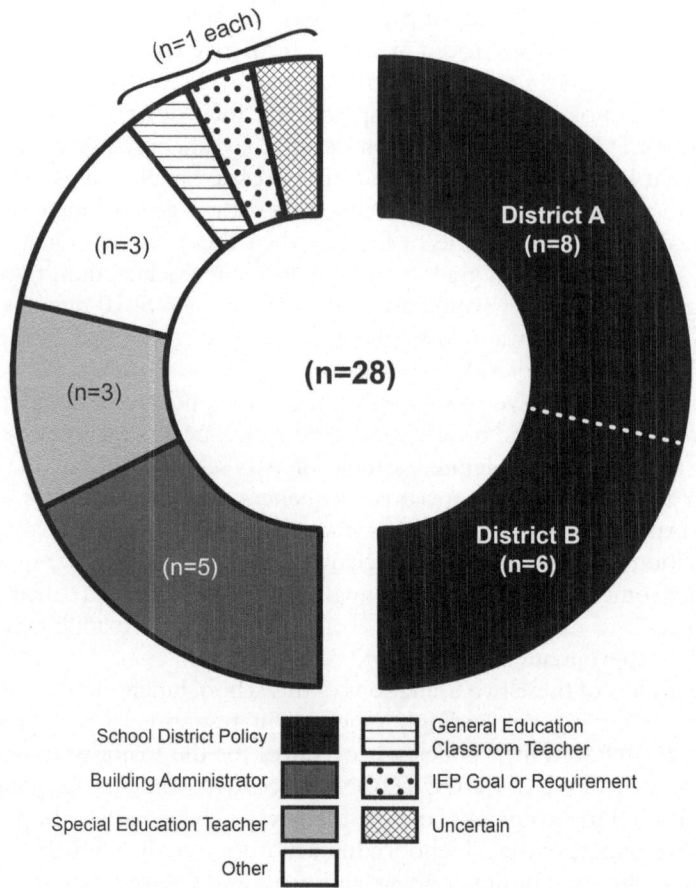

**Fig. 8.2**   Lunch policy and procedure determination: administrator responses

respondents ($n = 77$ of 224) answered that school lunch policy and procedures were "determined by school district policy." The remaining 147 non-administrator respondents provided one of the nine other answers (see Fig. 8.3).

Given the wide disparity of responses to the policy and procedures determination question, not only between administrators and non-administrators but also within each of these two groups, we reached out

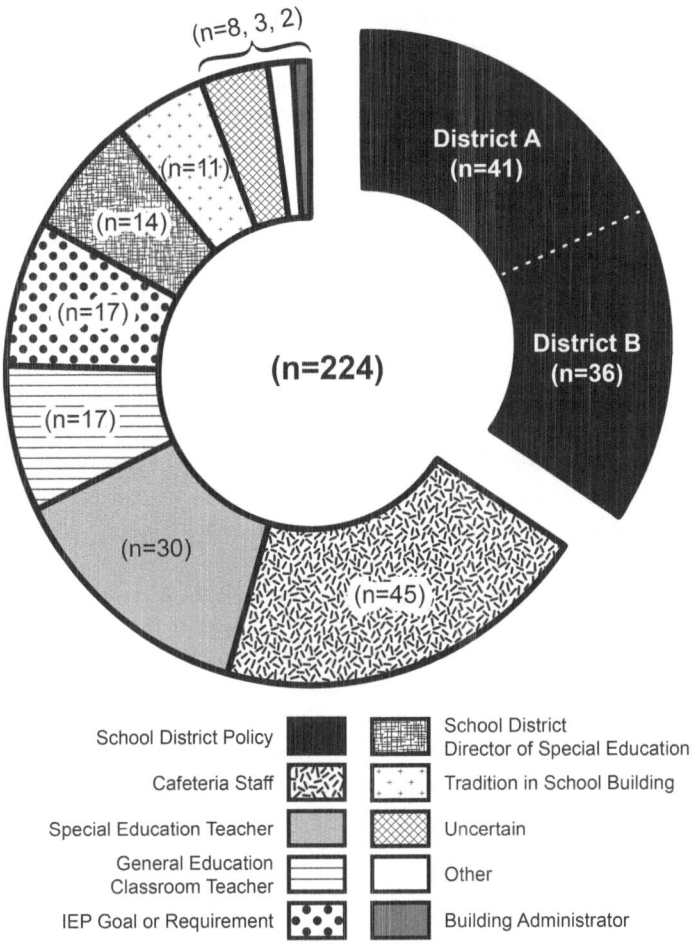

**Fig. 8.3** Lunch policy and procedure determination: non-administrator responses

to the Directors of Special Education of the two participating districts, seeking clarification. Through personal communication with the directors in District A (June 7, 2017) and District B (May 30, 2017), it was discovered that in *neither* district does either (1) school district policy or (2) procedures for addressing lunchroom practices for students who receive general or special education services exist in writing. It would appear that much work remains to be done in regard to the full inclusion of students who experience disabilities in school lunchrooms—but given the absence of obstructive school district policy to define daily practice and procedures, the opportunity for such change seems both timely and possible.

## THE FUTURE OF SCHOOL LUNCH PRACTICE

A few notable examples of current educational practice illustrate the attempt to foster a more welcoming environment in the school lunchroom. The non-profit Southern Poverty Law Center (2017), best known for tracking American hate groups, sponsors "Mix It Up at Lunch Day." Since 2002 the Center has designated the last Tuesday of October as "Mix It Up at Lunch Day." On this day, students are assigned lunch seatmates, students with whom they would not usually share a meal. The Center has a website with a variety of activities and resources addressing such issues as empathy, acceptance, and curtailing cliques. Schools can register, at no cost, to receive free materials and to connect with other participating schools through various social networking sites.

Ng et al. (2013) studied a program similar to "Mix It Up at Lunch Day" in one school setting with students in grades 6–12. Students in this school were randomly seated at tables in the lunchroom throughout the school year. Ng and colleagues concluded that the program they studied was "affirming and readily adaptable" (p. 76), and saw the program as "an illustration of what can be realized" if schools want to use lunchtime to promote greater inclusion among students (p. 76). In an elementary school setting, Heyne et al. (2012) implemented a "lunch bunch program" to support interactions and relationships between students who experience disability and their typically developing peers. Through consultation with classroom teachers, groups of four to five students were assembled, one of whom experienced disability. Based on the success of their efforts, these researchers, suggest that educational teams give more consideration to formally structuring lunch (and recess) programs to facilitate the development of friendships between these groups of young students.

These examples illustrate how structured, intentional programs and procedures can facilitate positive change in school lunchrooms. Yet for researchers, families, practitioners, administrators, and policy-makers, the questions remain: What is the current practice in school lunchrooms? Who determines the procedures to be followed? What formal policy determines practice and procedures implemented? How can structure and practice help in cultivating a richer sense of interconnectedness among students who receive special education services and their typically developing peers? With the relatively recent call to examine the social consequences of school lunch (Weaver-Hightower 2011), the lack of attention to the lunchroom experiences of students who receive special education services is both curious and problematic. The lunchroom as a space with important social concerns for students who receive special education services should be examined more thoughtfully and systematically. Such examination should include the policies and practices governing the lunchroom as well as the actual lunchroom social interactions involving this student population. Significant social encounters transpire during lunch, each school day, for students across the United States and the world. It is imperative to begin to focus on those who are particularly vulnerable to their consequences.

## NOTE

1. The authors of this chapter have retained the language used at the time a referenced study was conducted or a paper written. In no current context is the term "mental retardation" appropriate or endorsed by these writers.

## REFERENCES

Eckert, P. (1989). *Jocks and burnouts: Social categories and identity in high school.* New York: Columbia University, Teachers College.

Eder, D. (1995). *School talk: Gender and adolescent culture.* New Brunswick: Rutgers University.

Furlow, T. W. (1973). A matter of life and death. *Pharos, 36*(3), 84–90.

Gargiulo, R. M., & Bouck, E. C. (2018). *Special education in contemporary society: An introduction to exceptionality* (6th ed.). Los Angeles: Sage.

Hallahan, D. P., Kauffman, J. M., & Pullen, P. C. (2015). *Exceptional learners: An introduction to special education* (13th ed.). Boston: Pearson.

Heyne, L., Wilkins, V., & Anderson, L. (2012). Social inclusion in the lunchroom and on the playground at school. *Social Advocacy and Systems Change Journal, 3*(1), 54–68.

*Individuals with Disabilities Education Improvement Act of 2004 (IDEA),* 20 U.S.C. §1400 et seq.

Kanner, L. (1964). *A history of the care and study of the mentally retarded.* Springfield: Charles C. Thomas.

Kunc, N. (1992). *The need to belong: Rediscovering Maslow's hierarchy of needs*. Retrieved from http://www.broadreachtraining.com/articles/armaslow.htm

Kunc, N. (1995). *The other side of therapy: Disability, normalcy, and the tyranny of rehabilitation*. Retrieved from Axis Consultation & Training, Ltd., November 4, 2004. http://www.normemma.com

Kunc, N., & Van der Klift, E. (1995). *A credo for support*. Retrieved from http://www2.gnb.ca/content/dam/gnb/Departments/pcsdp-cpmcph/pdf/docs/CredoforSupport.pdf

Lauer, V. K. (2014). *When the school says no...how to get the yes! Securing special education services for your child*. London: Jessica Kingsley.

Levine, S. (2008). *School lunch politics: The surprising history of America's favorite welfare program*. Princeton: Princeton University.

Maslow, A. (1970). *Motivation and personality* (2nd ed.). New York: Harper & Row.

McKnight, J. (1995). *The careless society: Community and its counterfeits*. New York: BasicBooks, Perseus.

Milner, M. (2004). *Freaks, geeks, and cool kids: American teenagers, schools, and the culture of consumption*. London: Routledge.

National Center for Education Statistics, Institute of Education Sciences. (2009). *Characteristics of public school districts in the United States: Results from the 2007–08 schools and staffing survey. First look*. Retrieved from https://nces.ed.gov/pubs2009/2009320.pdf

Ng, J., Sweeney, H. M., & Mitchiner, M. (2013). Let's sit together: Exploring the potential for human relations education at lunch. *Journal of Thought, 48*(2), 65–77.

Perske, R. (1991). *Unequal justice? What can happen when persons with retardation or other developmental disabilities encounter the criminal justice system*. Nashville: Abingdon.

President's Committee on Mental Retardation. (1970). *The six-hour retarded child*. Washington, DC: Author.

Smith, J. D. (1995). *Pieces of purgatory: Mental retardation in and out of institutions*. Pacific Grove: Brookes/Cole.

Smith, J. D., & Wehmeyer, M. L. (2012). *Good blood bad blood: Science, nature, and the myth of the Kallikaks*. Washington, DC: American Association on Intellectual and Developmental Disabilities.

Southern Poverty Law Center. (2017). *Teaching tolerance*. Retrieved March 6, 2017, from http://www.tolerance.org/mix-it-up/what-is-mix

Tatum, B. D. (1997). *Why are all the Black kids sitting together in the cafeteria? And other conversations about race*. New York: BasicBooks.

Thorne, B. (1993). *Gender play: Girls and boys in school*. New Brunswick: Rutgers University.

Turnbull, A., Turnbull, R., Wehmeyer, M. L., & Shogren, K. A. (2016). *Exceptional lives: Special education in today's schools* (8th ed.). Boston: Pearson.

Weaver-Hightower, M. B. (2011). Why education researchers should take school food seriously. *Educational Researcher, 40,* 15–21.

# CHAPTER 9

# School Lunch and Student Food Insecurity: A Teacher's Observations and Reflections

*Sarah Riggs Stapleton and Person Cole*

## INTRODUCTION

While critical educators consider the ways in which students from low-income families, many of whom are of color, experience oppression and marginalization in and through schooling, seldom do they focus on the food students are offered at school. For formal educators, food in schools is ever present yet underexamined (Weaver-Hightower 2011). The percentage of students qualifying for free or reduced-fee lunch is used by educators as a proxy indicator of the socioeconomic status of school communities. However, formal educators' considerations of school lunch typically end at citing statistics. Given the extent to which school lunches impact the lives, health, cultural identities, and well-being of our most vulnerable students, it is a significant oversight that we neglect to critically examine the food our students are being served in schools as part of the school curriculum.

Robert and Weaver-Hightower (2011a) have argued that food has been ignored in education (as well as the humanities and social sciences)

S. R. Stapleton (✉)
University of Oregon, Eugene, OR, USA

P. Cole
Alternative High School, Michigan, USA

© The Author(s) 2018
S. Rice, A. G. Rud (eds.), *Educational Dimensions of School Lunch*,
https://doi.org/10.1007/978-3-319-72517-8_9

157

because it falls on the wrong side of the mind-body dualism split, being relegated to the body rather than the mind. Far from being an issue separate from education, Robert and Weaver-Hightower (2011a) argue that "food practices are a means of social reproduction, oppression, and resistance" (p. 17), noting that "for educators, researchers, and policymakers, this requires viewing school food as one of the central facets of school reform" (p. 16).

While efforts to improve school lunches have occurred, these have mostly arisen from non-educators outside of schools. Interestingly, the history of school food provides more context on why this aspect of the curriculum has fallen outside the purview of formal educators. School meals began in the Progressive Era prior to World War I and, at that time, fell under the jurisdiction of charities, women's groups, PTAs, and other non-educators (Levine 2008; Poppendieck 2010). This trend continues with concerns about school lunches being voiced primarily by celebrities, celebrity chefs, parents, activists, and non-formal educators (e.g. "Renegade Lunch Lady" Chef Ann Cooper, Alice Waters, Michelle Obama, FoodCorps). While this is important work (and we clearly need all hands on deck), we have argued (Stapleton et al. 2017) that formal educators working in schools on a daily basis bring needed perspectives to the issue. Teachers, in particular, have key placements within schools, and in relation to students, that can enable them to see and ask critical questions on food issues faced by their students.

It is no secret that the quality of school food is low. A singular word— "nasty"—has been uttered by countless people when asked to describe their school lunches (Poppendieck 2010). While the quality of school food in and of itself is an important issue to address for the sake of *all* kids in schools, in this chapter, we are turning special attention to students who are food insecure. By food insecure, we mean that they do not have consistent and reliable access to food in their lives outside of schools. Giving food-insecure students access to free/reduced-price lunches is an important, ethical act as it may be the only reliable access to food each day for youth in approximately 3 million US households (USDA Economic Research Service 2016). There have been strides under The Healthy, Hunger-Free Kids Act of 2010 to increase access to food in schools, through the Community Eligibility Provision (CEP) which allows high-poverty schools to provide free meals to all with no need for family applications. While this is an important step, we demonstrate here why it is not enough.

In this chapter, we take a food justice approach: we consider access to high-quality, nutritious, tasty, and culturally sustaining food in schools as a right for all students. Our food justice perspective brings attention to social injustice along the lines of race and class to the food movement arena and is informed by scholars such as Alkon and Agyeman (2011). Following this, we bring terms from the food justice world such as food insecurity and food deserts into the school food arena. While we are very much in support of food movements that advocate for local, organic, and equitably sourced food for animals and people, in this chapter, we focus on three areas regarding school food: quality, nutrition, and cultural relevance. In our work, we share a veteran teacher's insights about food insecurity as experienced by her students. Based on her observations, we introduce the idea of *in-school food insecurity*, the situation in which students choose not to eat school food despite being food insecure *and* having universally free access to school food. We consider factors that can increase or decrease students' in-school food insecurity and suggest ways to account more accurately for whether or not students are facing in-school food insecurity.

## SITUATING THE PROJECT AND THE AUTHORS

The ideas presented in this chapter stem from a participatory action research project with teachers which Sarah, an education researcher, led as part of her doctoral dissertation work (Stapleton 2015a). Sarah is a white woman who has lived all over the United States and internationally. She is a former middle/high school teacher and current teacher educator and seeks to engage teachers as collaborators in research. The goal of her dissertation project was to encourage teachers to focus (broadly) on food issues in schools within a low-income, urban school district in the Midwest and share their perspectives from their positions as teachers.

Person was one of four teachers who participated as partners in the project. She and Sarah met at a local food justice conference, where they discovered their shared passions around food justice for students. Person has spent 38 years working as a special education teacher in a low-income school district in a Midwestern city. She is an African American woman, who grew up in another urban center in the same state. Based on her extensive experience teaching in the same school district for decades, she is highly knowledgeable about the city, school district, local/regional politics, and local/regional demographics. That Person's own childhood was marked by hunger shapes how she thinks about food security for her students and explains her attentiveness to it. Her history and experiences make her perspective particularly persuasive and authentic. She reflects:

> The issue of food security in my urban center has caused me to do a lot of soul searching and thinking. As a child growing up in the '60s, I was very aware of no food, lack of food, being hungry, and not knowing what I could do about it. Now I'm well past childhood and I still have that sense of food insecurity and concern about a lack of food for urban kids.

Person's awareness of the importance of food security sparked her to question food insecurity at her school. To do this, she made observations of school lunches and students' eating patterns during the school day. She interviewed the school food coordinator about the systems and procedures for feeding students. She witnessed the meals being served, and whether students were eating. She also talked with students about their opinions on the food at various times of the lunch period. She also observed the vending machine sales each week, noting how much of what items were being purchased. Within the period in which Person was engaged in her study (the 2013–14 and 2014–15 school years) the district changed contracts, hiring a new food service provider. Interestingly, Person witnessed a noticeable change in food quality across the two years. Person's written account is shared in the following sections. Her words and observations are in italics so that her voice is distinguishable. After Person's observations are shared, Sarah discusses how Person's observations speak to literature on food and school food.

## FOOD INSECURITY AT AN ALTERNATIVE HIGH SCHOOL

*I [Person] work at an alternative high school (AHS), where we specialize in working with at-risk students. I have worked with this population for over 15 years. My school is not in a traditional school with access to a kitchen, so the food is pre-packaged so that it can be heated in an industrial oven. The food is "bussed" in, and the students eat from elementary-like foam trays.*

*From our school improvement report, our documented free and reduced lunch rate is 97%. Everybody in our school gets to eat for free. And you would think that since everybody gets to eat free, they would come and eat. But they don't.*

*"Ms. Cole, I'm hungry."*
*"Why don't you get lunch?"*
*"I'm not eating that food."*
*"Oh, so you'd rather go to the vending machines?"*
*"Yes, because I'm not eating that food."*

*The at-risk students I work with do have access to food through the free breakfast and lunch program, but the food quality has been less than ideal. The food choices in my school over the last 15 years have been foods that lead directly to obesity, diabetes, high blood pressure, and a host of other destructive health issues. My students get 97% processed food, white flour-based breads, canned fruits, and sometimes apples, oranges, and bananas as fresh fruit. Access to quality food is extremely limited. To add insult to injury, we have one vending machine with snacks and one vending machine with pop.*

*AHS is located in a food desert. The closest grocery store is 2 and ¼ miles away from the school, and this is in a community where there are a lot of people. Where the school is, there are five apartment complexes on just one side of the road. So it's not easy to get fresh fruits and vegetables there. My students get hungry, and they want food. But they don't know how to easily get it, and there's not a place for them to easily get it.*

*My school does not have access to the food that the other high schools have, which means that the most marginalized students in the district have the least access to good food. If a food desert in an urban setting is a place with limited access to fresh food/quality food, then my school [itself] is a food desert.*

\* \* \*

Person's observations are powerful for several reasons. First, Person identifies that within school districts there can be schools that have lesser quality food because of a lack of on-site kitchen facilities. Schools with lesser or no kitchen facilities have been of concern for years. In fact, Levine (2008) reports that it was this situation which ushered in the use of food service management corporations in 1969. Alarmingly, with the increasing rise of pre-packed foods, there are **new** schools being designed and built with no kitchen facilities, only "warming centers" for heating food prepared off-site (Kitchens without Cooks n.d.).

Person points to food security for students *within* the school day as a serious issue: food-insecure students—those who did not have reliable and/or adequate access to food at home—refusing to eat the food served by the school because it was of such poor quality. She even notes that her school *itself* could be considered a food desert. Through this statement, she applies food justice language to school food. By doing so, she brings two distinct food practice communities into dialogue, to foster social justice within school food practices. That a school *itself* can be a food desert is an important and powerful assertion and one which educators and school food decision makers should take seriously.

While several books consider issues of school food access to low-income students and the quality of school food (e.g. Levine 2008; Poppendieck 2010; Robert and Weaver-Hightower 2011a, b), none make the direct observation that students with ready access to free food may not eat it because of low quality. Much of the focus of existing school food literature concerns the *access* of students from low-income families to free food, as eligibility for free/reduced-price lunch status presents countless problems (e.g. Poppendieck 2010). An additional concern that appears in literature is the stigma associated with accepting free/reduced-price meals in schools serving students from heterogeneous social-economic backgrounds (Poppendieck 2010). It has been argued that an answer to these problems is to provide free meals for all (Poppendieck 2010). Because all students in Person's district are automatically eligible for free meals, Person's observations demonstrate that the solution is not that simple.

## THE SLIPPERINESS OF STUDENT HUNGER

*You don't ask high-risk children, "Do you get enough to eat?" You don't ask that because you've got a fight. You don't ask them, "Do you have enough food at home?" No, you don't ask high-risk children that—especially a teenager or young to late adolescent. There's the wall of pride and the wall of shame. And the wall of pride is huge—you can't get through that. And the wall of shame? You are not getting through that. Unless there is a deep, penetrating relationship, kids are not going to discuss food security. They're not.*

*Some of their parents will note when the mobile food pantry is going to be in their neighborhood. Near the school, there is a church with a monthly food drop. When mobile food pantries are going to be in my area, we usually get a flyer sent to us, and we're to tell the kids. You've got to be careful how you say it, like I said, that pride and that shame. You just can't go up to a kid and say, 'Hey, the mobile food truck 'gonna be in the neighborhood. Tell your ma.' We cannot do that. We post the information and make a general announcement. We don't single out anybody.*

*My children (my students) do not seem to understand the social implications of food security. When I gave them surveys using the term "food security," every student asked me what it meant. (I had never heard of food security myself until I went to a local food justice conference.) They're disconnected from their lack of food, the causes, and what they can do themselves to solve the problem. This situation keeps them confined and perpetuates the continuation of food insecurity for them. It's cyclical.*

\* \* \*

As someone who experienced hunger as a student but was forbidden by her mother to accept free food from her school, Person is aware of the nuances and challenges of understanding individual students' food security. Person's testimony points to how complicated it can be to try to get at food insecurity in schools and for individual students, even as someone who grew up in similar circumstances. Her awareness points to the importance of finding other measures (such as observing students at lunch) rather than asking students directly to investigate student hunger. Because her school has a 97% free and reduced-rate lunch, we can be fairly certain that nearly all students are in need of food, which makes this an ideal case study for this work.

Person also points to her students not being aware of the larger systemic food situation in which they are nested and trapped. This lack of awareness speaks to the need for educators to teach about food justice issues in their classrooms so that students have exposure to food justice language and concepts and might apply them to their lives.

## THE IMPACT OF FOOD SERVICE MANAGEMENT CORPORATIONS

*When we first started this project, the district was still working with the company [name redacted at publisher request]. [The food service company] treated delivering food to my school as if it were an elementary school, sending so little it seemed like food rationing. There was no variety, and there was a limited amount of food. Students complained about the terrible food. It was horrible.*

*The following year, when a new food company came in, they brought in more variety and more food. The daily standard food is a spicy chicken patty (which the children love), a regular chicken patty, and chicken nuggets. Even though the kids still have spicy chicken patties, they can get two spicy chicken patties if they like. Last year they never served fish, but now during Lent, they serve fish once a week and the fish patties are of nice quality. The variety is exciting; there is corn on the cob, potato wedges made from real potatoes, and baked fried chicken once or twice a week. The baked fried chicken looks fried, but it's baked. They even have baked-fried drumsticks; you don't have to ask if it's chicken. ... [The former food service company] never served anything like that.*

*[The new company] has brought in more variety for the kids, more food for the kids, so more kids are now eating. I find that fascinating. I don't hear the kids complaining...They complained a lot [when the previous company was there], but now I'm not hearing complaints. So, to answer the question, "If you serve better food, will more kids eat?" I'm going to go with "yes," especially if the food is familiar to them. There has been a change in food security for our students. This new company provides a larger variety, and the kids notice it, like it, and they're eating. I'm excited about that.*

*[The new company] has provided food for the afternoon kids who go to school from 1–5 pm whereas last year, the afternoon students didn't have any food. Last year, to supplement the afternoon students, the teachers would bring in crackers and snack pretzels, and one of the teachers would request at least ten milks. Now, there is a whole hot box with food for at least 30 kids, and in the afternoon at 3:30 pm, there's a line...When they leave the school, if they got food at 3:30 pm, then they've got something in their belly, and they can wait until the next day.*

\* \* \*

It was perhaps a serendipitous occurrence that Person's project timeline coincided with the changing of the food services contract in her district, allowing her to observe the impacts of this change on student food consumption. The dramatic and instantaneous shift in school lunch quality from one school year to the next is startling. It is important to note that this change also coincided with the enactment in 2014 of *The Healthy, Hunger-Free Kids Act*, and could also (or otherwise) have been connected to changes in the language used in the district's request for food service proposals. While the exact causes of this change are beyond the scope of this research project, it is nonetheless fascinating to note that the changes did not result from a systemic overhaul of the district's food service system.

In looking at Person's narrative, there are some key phrases worth examining. That the initial food service company's meals appeared to Person as "food rationing" is one such phrase, connoting conditions of scarcity as in war or punishment. As part of this, Person has questioned the practice that her high school students—including groups with particularly high caloric needs like teenage boys and pregnant young women—have been served the same amount as the youngest elementary students in the district. I [Sarah] will add here my concern that *The Healthy, Hunger-Free Kids Act* reduces portion sizes for youth. I recognize that this is an attempt to address obesity, but students—especially those in high school—are growing and have higher caloric needs than later in life. It is important to note that childhood obesity may be as connected (if not more) to the composition of foods (highly processed, high in sugar, fat) rather than the quantity alone. Moreover, childhood obesity is highly correlated with low income, not because children are eating too much per se, but because the foods that are most commonly available to their families (who disproportionately live in food deserts) are typically highly processed and nutrient poor. For these reasons, I advocate the unlimited availability of nutrient-dense food rather than limiting portion size as an ethical practice for food-insecure youth.

It seems important to call out food service companies for low-quality food as an unethical practice, particularly for its impact on food-insecure students. (That said, we were prohibited by the publisher from including the name of the company whose service was terrible.) Around this time, the intial food service company received substantial negative publicity in the state for its involvement with a prison food scandal. (It is unclear, however, how much this scandal impacted the district's decision to create a contract with another company.). Publicity about the company's low-quality food is continually emerging, such as a 2016 boycott staged by some Chicago Public School high school students and their teacher, Tim Meegan (Eng 2015, Nov 30; Perkins 2016, Feb 4). These students and their teacher specifically objected to the low-quality of their school food, calling out brown lettuce, gray broccoli, served-but-still-frozen food (Eng 2015, Nov 30; Perkins 2016, Feb 4). This company's food controversies are not limited to K-12 schools, but have also extended to colleges and prison scandals (e.g. Zoukis 2015, Dec 2).

Poppendieck (2010) recognizes that student participation (receiving of a school lunch) can change slightly by food service staff "branding" lunchrooms, bringing in new dishes, revamping their image, and so on. However, the significance of a local decision made, often haphazardly, by a district school board for addressing (or not addressing) student food insecurity needs far more attention in the literature.

## IMPORTANCE OF CULTURAL RECOGNITION OF STUDENTS THROUGH FOOD

*Food programs do not [but should] take into account the ethnicity of food, the diversity of food. On February 1, 2015, the new company served kids rib tips with real barbecue sauce, collard greens, cornbread muffins, and sautéed apples. When the company served these foods in our predominantly African American school, there wasn't anything left. When one child saw another's plate, they'd ask, "Where did you get that?" More and more kids who normally don't want to eat were eating. Some asked, "Are y'all doing this for black history month?"*

\* \* \*

In her historical exploration of school food, Levine (2008) points out that early on, with the advent of nutrition science, school lunches were a platform for "Americanizing" the diet of immigrant children living in the United States. In other words, not only were school lunches inattentive to the highly diverse backgrounds of American students early on, they were intentionally tone deaf to culturally responsive feeding. Moreover, dietary recommendations created and made official by the US Department of Agriculture, further institutionalized cultural imperialism through school lunches (Levine 2008) as they were based on a dominant-culture diet.

The importance of students having access to culturally appropriate foods cannot be underemphasized for the key role that food plays in shaping, expressing, and cultivating identity (e.g. Bell and Valentine 1997; Caplan 1997; Greene and Cramer 2011; Stapleton 2015b). Robert and Weaver-Hightower (2011a, b) argue that school food is a window into identity and culture as "food establishes who we are in gendered, sexualized, raced, and ethnic senses, and who we are through food has social consequences" (p. 14). Food plays an important role in expressing who we are to others and in supporting group identities (Stapleton 2015b). Since schools are public spaces where students are encountered and interacting with others from many different food cultures, school food plays a role in sustaining/not sustaining or validating/invalidating students' cultural foods.

## How We "Check" Boxes

*I think the school food coordinator does a phenomenal job in addressing the issue of food security with our students. She has been working with me on this project. The district wasn't going to send us enough food because we accept children out of the district (because it's an alternative program, and we have all kinds of special programs). The district keeps careful records of all food distributed. But the food coordinator has her own system. When she makes a plate, she records a hashmark and counts all the sides for that plate, even if someone asks for just one item (so sides are left over, but they are counted as being used). If they send over 100 broccoli packages, for example, she may give out 60 broccoli packages, so 40 broccoli packages are left. But, instead of giving back the extras, she serves them to the afternoon students. Then she can tell the district, I went through 100 in a day, so I need 100 tomorrow, too. That's how she feeds the afternoon kids. I think she is being wise. She's demonstrating that there's not waste.*

*She's also creative in her food presentation and in getting food into the kids. When she serves nachos, she always puts a little extra something on them. She orders jalapeños and sour cream, and when she makes the nachos, the kids just love how she puts that together. She also insists that the kids get a vegetable.*

*[The new food service company] now prepackages their servings of fruit and vegetables. So, half an apple is a serving and they cut it already in their packaging. The lunch coordinator gives it to them and tells them they can throw it in their backpack. It's wonderful.*

\* \* \*

There are a number of important points presented in Person's reflections here. First, while all the students in the district are provided free meals, students from outside the district (who may be just as food insecure) are not accommodated because of the way school districts are delineated and budgeted. In other words, food-insecure students served by special programs can get caught in between district accounting systems.

Second, Person's observations point to the importance of a single food service staff member for increasing food security. She illustrates that much—in this case beating accounting systems to acquire more food and making the food more enticing—depends on the initiative of individuals within the system. After Person articulated these thoughts, the food service director took a leave of absence due to family emergency. With her absence, Person saw the quality of food drop immediately. Even after receiving a replacement food service staff member, Person observed that the food amount and quality continued to decrease.

Person's selection of the preposition "getting food *into* kids" is an important choice. Given all the observations Person has shared, this occurrence should not be underestimated, as we argue that in-school food insecurity arises primarily because students are not ingesting food, even when it is freely accessible to them. This situation points to the inadequacy of the way current boxes are checked to "show" that kids are being fed in schools. Rather than simply checking boxes that kids were given food, we must attend to real measures that accurately portray what students are actually eating.

## ASKING CRITICAL QUESTIONS

*Food security is [a] very complex issue and even though there are grassroots efforts to try to remedy food security in general, I'm left with these questions: Who is in the grassroots? Where is the grassroots work being done, and to benefit whom?*

By questioning *who* gets to make decisions around school food and *to what end* they are collecting data about who is given food (rather than about the rates at which food is consumed), Person has articulated important concerns about what it means to feed food-insecure students in schools. Her sentiment is echoed by Sandler (2011) who argues that we need to ask the following critical questions of school feeding: "Who feeds whom what, how, and for what purpose?" (p. 33). Both Person's and Sandler's (2011) questions encourage us to think more ethically in our approach to school feeding.

## SOME ALTERNATIVES FOR MEASURING IN-SCHOOL FOOD SECURITY

Person has exposed the gaping problems in the way we account for feeding the youth in schools. Through her observations, we see that merely measuring when students are given food does not even come close to the type of accounting we need to accurately determine whether or not we are preventing in-school food insecurity among students.

If our aims are to ameliorate in-school food insecurity, perhaps we need to change the way we do our accounting. This suggests that we may need to "check" boxes based on whether or not the students are *actually eating food.*

**Food Waste** One idea is to measure the food waste being created each day as it will indicate how much food is consumed versus thrown away. If students are asked to sort their garbage, separating out the food, this can also help schools move toward environmentally sustainable practices like composting.

**Student Satisfaction** Another idea is to survey students regularly about whether or not they are eating and how they feel about the food. With a plethora of options to survey students using cell phone technologies, tablets, and so on, this could be an easy, stream-lined daily process.

**Parent Satisfaction** While parents are sometimes a little far removed from knowing exactly what their children are consuming each day, parents may still be an important source of information about how well a school food program is meeting the needs of its community. Parents are perhaps the most concerned members about the quality of food their children are receiving, so it is important to keep them in the loop.

## CONCLUDING THOUGHTS

As formal educators, we have cultivated an ability to ignore the significance and implications of food served in schools for our students. While we worry about the hidden curriculum in other aspects of the school day, we are blind when it comes to school food. The authors have argued that those interested in food justice in schools should partner with formal educators as insiders in school systems (Stapleton et al. 2017). More specifically, this chapter has argued that formal educators should focus explicitly on the role that food in schools plays in supporting (or not supporting) low-income, marginalized students. Person's observations reveal that feeding food-insecure kids in schools can be surprisingly precarious— both dependent on a district's contract agreements with food service management companies and on an individual staff member's prowess.

In reflecting on the tremendous and direct consequences that food service management corporations have on student food insecurity, ideally, we would extricate corporations from the US school lunch scene. However, if we can only take small steps, Person's observations suggest that it is possible for these corporations to do better (and worse), and that by increasing the quality of the food served, the problem of in-school food insecurity for students may be reduced. Despite strides made under the Obama administration to improve school food quality and access, with a new administration the political winds have changed, and the already-inadequate federal funding of free and reduced-fee lunches may be in jeopardy (Jalonick May 2017). Given this hostile political climate, there is even greater need for teachers to include school food in their purview and to look out particularly for students who are food insecure. As educators we must not be blind to our students' most basic and important need: food. Given the ways in which food is inextricably linked to identity (Stapleton 2015b), we must recognize the message that low-quality school food transmits to our kids about their worth and join the fight to improve it.

## REFERENCES

Alkon, A. H., & Agyeman, J. (Eds.). (2011). *Cultivating food justice: Race, class, and sustainability.* Cambridge, MA: MIT Press.

Bell, D., & Valentine, G. (1997). *Consuming geographies: We are where we eat.* London: Routledge.

Caplan, P. (1997). Approaches to the study of food, health and identity. In P. Caplan (Ed.), *Food, health and identity* (pp. 1–31). London: Routledge.

Eng, M. (2015, November 30). *Chicago high schoolers launch website against school food.* WBEZ 91.5 Chicago News. https://www.wbez.org/shows/wbez-news/chicago-high-schoolers-launch-website-against-school-food/eafe13ae-882d-472f-9da9-0bd876778137. Accessed 4/5/17.

Greene, C. P., & Cramer, J. M. (2011). Beyond mere sustenance: Food as communication/communication as food. In J. M. Cramer, C. P. Greene, & L. M. Walters (Eds.), *Food as communication, communication as food* (pp. iv–xix). New York: Peter Lang Publishing.

Jalonick, M. (2017, May 1). *Trump administration to cut some school lunch standards.* US News and World Reports. Accessed from: https://www.usnews.com/news/news/articles/2017-05-01/agriculture-to-roll-back-some-standards-on-school-meals

Kitchens without cooks: A future of frozen food for Chicago's schoolchildren? (n.d.). A report by Unite Here & Let's Cook organizations. http://www.realfoodrealjobs.org/wp-content/uploads/UNITE-HERE-Kitchens-Without-Cooks-_-FINAL.pdf. Accessed 4/5/17.

Levine, S. (2008). *School lunch politics: The surprising history of America's favorite welfare program.* Princeton: Princeton University Press.

Perkins, T. (2016, February 4). *How Chicago students are fighting disgusting school lunches.* Vice. https://munchies.vice.com/en_us/article/how-chicago-students-are-fighting-disgusting-school-lunches. Accessed 4/5/17.

Poppendieck, J. (2010). *Free for all: Fixing school food in America.* Berkeley: University of California Press.

Robert, S., & Weaver-Hightower, M. (2011a). Introduction. In S. Robert & M. Weaver-Hightower (Eds.), *School food politics* (pp. 201–208). New York: Peter Lang.

Robert, S., & Weaver-Hightower, M. (2011b). Coda: Healthier horizons. In S. Robert & M. Weaver-Hightower (Eds.), *School food politics* (pp. 201–208). New York: Peter Lang.

Sandler, J. (2011). Reframing the politics of urban feeding in the U.S. public schools: Parents, programs, activists, and the state. In S. Robert & M. Weaver-Hightower (Eds.), *School food politics* (pp. 25–45). New York: Peter Lang.

Stapleton, S. R. (2015a). Teacher participatory action research on food insecurity, food and culture, and school gardens within a low-income urban school district (Doctoral dissertation). Retrieved from Michigan State University.

Stapleton, S. R. (2015b). Food, identity, & environmental education. *Canadian Journal of Environmental Education, 20,* 12–24.

Stapleton, S. R., Alvarado, T., Cole, P., Jason, M., & Washburn, M. (2017). Views from the classroom: Teachers on food in a low-income urban school district. In I. Werkheiser & Z. Piso (Eds.), *Food justice in US and global contexts: Bringing theory and practice together* (pp. 129–140). New York: Springer.

USDA Economic Research Service. (2016, October 11). *Key statistics and graphics.* Accessed from: https://www.ers.usda.gov/topics/food-nutrition-assistance/food-security-in-the-us/key-statistics-graphics.aspx

Weaver-Hightower, M. (2011). Why education researchers should take school food seriously. *Educational Researcher, 40*(1), 15–21.

Zoukis, C. (2015, Dec 2). *Aramark's correctional food services: Meals, maggots, and misconduct.* Prison Legal News. https://www.prisonlegalnews.org/news/2015/dec/2/aramarks-correctional-food-services-meals-maggots-and-misconduct/. Accessed 4/5/17.

# CHAPTER 10

# School Lunch Curriculum

## *A. G. Rud and Shannon Gleason*

Eating during the midday at school has evolved from the time of the first public schools in the USA in the nineteenth century. There is evidence of isolated efforts to provide lunch at school starting as early as the mid-1800s. But this practice is generally traced to the Progressive Era. In large cities such as New York, Boston, and Philadelphia, among others, lunch programs were instituted out of concern about the nutrition of poor children attending urban schools, but also in an effort to Americanize immigrant school children (Levenstein 1988, 1993; Ziegelman 2010). At school, youngsters were encouraged to develop American tastes and habits—literally in the lunchroom—as foods native to their home countries were replaced with what was at the time standard American fare. Public school lunches were formally institutionalized in 1946 with the passage of the Richard B. Russell National School Lunch Act. Fast forward to the 1980s, and school lunch began to educate tastes in quite another way, as soft drink and fast food companies started selling their products in schools. Sugary drinks and fried food, once "treats" to be enjoyed occasionally, became integral to the everyday diet of many young people. We tend to think of school lunch as an activity occurring in, well,

A. G. Rud (✉)
Washington State University, Pullman, WA, USA

S. Gleason
Westfield State University, Westfield, MA, USA

© The Author(s) 2018
S. Rice, A. G. Rud (eds.), *Educational Dimensions of School Lunch*,
https://doi.org/10.1007/978-3-319-72517-8_10

school. Most students *do* consume their noontime meal within a school building, typically, within a cafeteria. Other student populations are generally overlooked in the school lunch literature: those who are educated at home, or "homeschooled," and those—almost always high schoolers—who dine off campus.

Most academic discussion of school food centers on nutritional content (e.g., Terry-McElrath et al. 2015), effects of school food on student health (e.g., Clark and Fox 2009), how to encourage healthier choices in school food (e.g., Miller et al. 2016; Zellner and Cobuzzi 2016), and assessments of the impact of school lunch programs on household food security (e.g., Arteaga and Heflin 2014; Huang and Barnidge 2016). Aside from this, there is a growing body of literature investigating the politics and social reality of school food (e.g., DeLeon 2011; Poppendieck 2013; Rowe and Rocha 2015; Rud 2013). In this book, authors have argued that school lunch is such an important part of the school day that it is essentially an informal yet explicit curriculum teaching students about food, the ethics of consumption, community, and the environment. As Rowe and Rocha (2015) state, school lunch is in fact an "overt, educational event" (p. 483). Rowe and Rocha (2015) argue that students are typically not conscious of school food as an educational phenomenon: "very little about the cafeteria-style lunch or the organization of schools and curricula enables students to know anything concerning the origins or actual constitution of their food" (p. 485). Further, while centered as objects of study, students are largely absent as agents in the school food discussion. In this chapter, we ask you to consider what it would look like to make school food a formal part of a school curriculum in which students would indeed learn about the origins, constitution, and politics of their lunch plate.

While school lunch has periodically been used for educational purposes throughout its history, it has usually been treated as an inconvenient necessity. In this chapter, we discuss some of the ways in which school lunch might be reconceived along more clearly educational lines. Specifically, we argue that a curriculum focusing upon school lunch as a component might provide an especially fruitful, structured opportunity to consider food consumed in a thoughtful way—where it comes from, how it is produced, and issues of nutrition and sustainability. The fact that school lunch is delivered in three distinctive ways makes conceptualizing such a curriculum rather challenging. Yet given the centrality of food in the individual and collective human experience, we believe that the effort is worthwhile.

School lunch, we suggest, is a hidden aspect of the explicit curriculum. How can we bring to theoretical light aspects of school lunch in order to begin to discern ways in which eating at midday might be theorized and integrated into a curriculum? We believe a more robust curriculum would view school lunch as an opportunity for inquiry into health, the body, and aspects of the good life that are not afforded through other kinds of classroom interaction. We use the work of John Dewey and Paulo Freire to aid us in theorizing school lunch. We conclude by offering a brief sketch of the philosophical basis of a curriculum that would include the consideration of school lunch in many of its manifestations.

## CHALLENGES TO MAKING SCHOOL LUNCH PART OF THE CURRICULUM

Our premise regarding the hidden curriculum of school lunch is that certain ways we have structured teaching and learning in the past and today influence how we look upon the meal of the midday. Furthermore, aspects of the hidden curriculum of schooling work toward how lunch is either a routine or an important part of the day.

In the school cafeteria paradigm, lunch is simply a part of the day that is not studied at all. It exists on the same plane as bathroom breaks or bus rides. Lunch is something that needs to be done midday but is not part of the instruction or co-curricular activities. In the case of homeschooling, one would think that there is a greater opportunity to treat lunch as a teaching moment. Yet even here, this moment is not taken advantage of in most circumstances. Research by A. G. Rud on midday eating for homeschoolers turned up mostly journalistic accounts of how busy moms make tasty sandwiches or fit instruction around the noon pit stop (Rud 2013). The teachers, usually mothers, do not treat lunch as part of the curriculum. Robert Kunzman's book about conservative Christian home schooling (2009) devotes little attention to school lunches for homeschoolers; lunch was not something expressly noted by the families he studied. For many parents teaching their children at home, lunch is a chore, at best. For the students who go off campus, it is possible that they could be alerted to concerns surrounding nutrition and sustainability that come up with eating out. Without adult intervention, this seems unlikely, and it is possible that many of these students have parents who are unaware of what their children are eating for lunch.

For homeschoolers, any conceptual understanding of the midday meal is limited by what the parents see as important for instruction. The prepackaged curricula many homeschoolers use leave little room for such discussion. It may be useful to request that the providers of these curricula consider a component on food preparation, nutrition, and cultural aspects of eating. In the case of open campus schools, there is little parental or adult supervision, and thus the opportunity for a curricular component to school lunch time is perhaps the most limited. Perhaps students could be encouraged to keep a food diary for nutrition or health classes or asked to collect images of fast food advertising for business or consumer literacy classes.

Food preparation and consumption should be an opportunity for learning. Otherwise, it becomes just part of the décor or what we do when we need to fill our stomachs. How this might be accomplished in any of these settings remains a difficult question. There are opportunities to learn from smaller experiments where children are involved in the cultivation of gardens and the preparation of foods, such as The Edible Schoolyard discussed by Susan Laird in her chapter (also see Laird 2008). Cafeteria-style school lunches in public schools remain part of the overall budget of that school, and thus are subject to budgetary pressures which may discourage innovation and connection to the broader curriculum. Even as cafeteria meals have become healthier in some schools, the opportunity to learn from them is limited. There are simply not many examples where lunch has been integrated into the curriculum.

A curriculum focusing upon school lunch should not be dependent upon these different instantiations of the midday meal. Two topics—nutrition and sustainability—could cut across cafeteria lunches, brown bags, parent-provided homeschool meals, or open campus restaurant options. For some students, this might be the only structured opportunity to consider the food—where it comes from, how it is produced, and issues of nutrition and sustainability. This would go a long way toward making school lunch an intentional, rather than an incidental, part of the curriculum and the school day.

## School Food Curriculum Rationale

With the disconnect between students and their school food in mind, we explored several approaches to building a school lunch curriculum and pedagogy, and ultimately identified two theoretical orientations from which such programs could draw. The first orientation is derived from John Dewey's philosophy of education, and uses a current example to illustrate Deweyan principles. The second is a Freirean-inspired popular education model, which emphasizes community-based reflection and action, and extends Dewey's approach to a more participatory level. These two radically democratic approaches could work in concert to make school lunch an intentional, rather than incidental, part of students' education. Further, a student-led centered focus on what, where, and how we consume and its effects on social and ecological justice would counter the emphasis on managerial, corporate, top-down—and often scripted—curriculum and pedagogy. Deweyan and Freirian perspectives are also outward looking; they do not simply offer care or concern for the Earth, but actively work toward producing a global citizenship and "authentic" solidarity (De Lissovoy 2010, p. 286) with all others and with the planet.

We make a case for considering John Dewey and Paulo Freire here in the context of school lunch by simply noting that whether at a school or at home, midday eating is a way for students to learn from the everyday and lift this relatively unexamined practice out of its place in daily routine and make it continuous with the rest of the school day. Thus, it becomes intentional and part of the day and not discontinuous and disconnected. School lunch can provide a unique occasion for learning that students cannot get in other areas. Let us first turn to how we can use John Dewey's thought to do this.

## DEWEY'S LEARNING BY DOING AND THE JOHN DEWEY KITCHEN INSTITUTE

To consider school lunch through Dewey's educational thought, we will describe the rationale of the John Dewey Kitchen Institute (JDKI) at the University of Vermont ("John Dewey Kitchen Institute" 2017). JDKI seeks to show ways that food is not only sustenance, but an occasion for learning. This is consistent with how Dewey viewed various kinds of activities and occupations, and instantiated them in the school he and his wife Alice ran at the University of Chicago. Children learned trades and arts as part of the school day.

The creators of JDKI show in some detail how the instructors integrate Deweyan insights and principles into a philosophy of food and consumption in an education for democracy. We list below their tenets ("JDKI

Tenets" 2017) and then discuss their relation to a Deweyan theoretical frame for school lunch.

The creators preface the tenets italicized below with a statement "The aim of education is the creation of a thriving democracy; the activity of education is itself an embodiment *of* democracy," and follow it with these tenets and explanations for a thoroughgoing link between Deweyan principles and a philosophy of food creation and consumption:

- Education as a Practice of Democracy: Education is democratic when it creates the possibility for growth in experience, the possibility for a better quality of human experience. You cannot do this alone. Thus, we teach and learn actively seeking to create democratic community.
- Education is Experience: Education is best understood as "intelligently directed development of the possibilities inherent in ordinary experience" (Experience and Education, Chapter 8). All experience is educative, but not all experience educates as we might desire; some experiences are mis-educative. (Experience and Education, Chapter 2) Thus, in the classroom, we create contexts that will foster genuinely educative experiences, that is, experiences that will promote further intellectual growth.
- Theory is Practice: The relationship between theory and practice is actually a relationship between two forms or modes of practice. When theory and practice operate together effectively, learners act reflectively and inquiringly, with a sense of purpose and for the sake of learning.
- Education begins with student experience and focuses on learning-the-activity, not learning-the-product: Learning happens best when it begins from students' experiences; when questions arise from them. Thus, we work to understand where students begin, what they know. Education emphasizes not things-learned (nouns), but learning (a verb). Learning emerges from experience, with a question or confusion. It leads to further experience. Thus, we seek to foster in students a capacity to ask the "next question" rather than to come up with "the right answer."
- Aims and Means Interact: A true aim, as opposed to one externally imposed, is something that will actually be a factor in choosing how one acts. True aims translate into means that a learner can understand, in which they can become engrossed, and which they can see

to the end. Thus, in teaching we work to enable students to identify and own their own aims.

- Play: Far from being trivial, play is "interested absorption in activity for the sake of activity itself" ("Growth in Activity"). Defined thus, it is the heart of education. As learners mature, this activity becomes more and more shaped by aims that are acknowledged, and even determined, by the learner. Thus, we treat play with serious respect, and make opportunities for it. Play can help to place children, *e.g.*, at the center of their education; the same can be true for adult learners.

- Chance and Change: Uncertainty is part of the fabric of our world, the fabric of our experience. Our interactions in the world must "live" with that fact. Thus, we aim to create in students the capacity to function flexibly in a world of chance and change.

- Nature-Culture: Nature and culture are deeply intertwined; humans are parts of nature. Human experience, human culture are thus both deeply natural and deeply cultural.

- Mind is a Verb: The human "mind" is not an organ, but a general character or attribute that infuses all of a human being, and draws upon the entirety of our bodies. To inquire, to investigate, to "mentally" explore our world always involves bodily engagement with that world. Thus, we create learning contexts that explicitly involve such engagement.

- Experience is "Double-Barreled": Human experiences are potentially either "instrumental" or "consummatory" or both; they lead us to a further experience, or they are enjoyed for their own sake. Education draws upon both kinds of experience.

These tenets give us a start to a Deweyan theoretical frame for school lunch, and some are more relevant to our purposes here than others. Midday eating is an experience from which we can learn, but it is also connected to the rest of schooling, and the various institutions (the family in the case of homeschooling, or the public or private school in the case of schooling outside the home) that participate in the educational enterprise. The distinction between theory and practice collapses in JDKI and can also do so if lunch is treated more intentionally as an educational experience connected to other such experiences in a school day. This would lead to what is said here about a focus on activity not product. Students could drill down into aspects of food production and consumption, and how each is connected to what they are learning in other parts of the curriculum.

While we endeavor to see midday eating as not simply caloric intake, but joined to other parts of the curriculum, it is an experience in itself, and has play and aesthetic aspects to it. Finally, perhaps more than anything other than play during recess time or physical education classes, midday eating deeply and obviously involves one's body. One can theorize about eating as we have done here, but it is an act of bodily engagement, not only to ingest food, but what that food is intended to do, both in satisfying hunger and providing essential nutrients to continue living. It is notable that the most understudied part of the day (midday eating) that we propose to be in the curriculum, is also at a fundamental level the most essential to sustaining learning.

## FREIRE AND POPULAR EDUCATION

As noted in other chapters of this book, school lunch is often decentered from the formal school curriculum, but has tremendous impact on students' daily, embodied experiences of schooling. Any school lunch curriculum ought to consider how to take the lived experiences of school children into account, while also encouraging the development of critical analysis and community action related to the food system, food (in)security, and school food. The idea of "popular education," with roots going back to the French Revolution, was also theorized as "conscientization" by Freire (2002) in *Pedagogy of the Oppressed*, and would be useful for this purpose. Popular education addresses student reality and values student agency in critically analyzing social institutions—such as school lunch—and organizing for social change. The meaning of "popular" in popular education stems from the notion that education is best led by "the people," especially the poor and working classes, in a community action where everyone teaches and everyone learns. Centering the student as agent, particularly considering the fact that students must actually consume food at school, would be key to a strong school food curriculum.

Popular education holds that all participants, especially and including students, possess expert knowledge about themselves, their communities, and the issues that affect them. Student knowledge is privileged by taking a bottom-up approach. Teachers, then, act as facilitators and collaborators to help expand and enable student knowledge and action. For a school food curriculum, this would mean that students could investigate not only the larger reality of US and global food systems, but also the local context of their own communities. What investigative work, for example, could students do to understand how their school food arrives on their plate? Could we lead them to ask who harvests, processes, prepares, and serves their food? Could they learn about and interrogate the social, economic, ecological, and cultural realities that effect these events? What kinds of inquiries could be made into students' own experiences of eating (or not) of food at school? What kind of intergenerational, historical knowledge could be tapped into if students engage with their families and other community elders about their own knowledge of food in and outside of school? These and other questions are expressly political in that there is an emphasis on understanding the class-, race-, gender-, religion-, and ability-based inequalities that are a major factor in who eats what, when, and how at school.

The learning community could not only ask these types of questions, and reflect on their collective, contextual knowledge of their actual lived experience, but could then act upon such knowledge to achieve change that positively affects the most vulnerable and marginalized (this can include both human and non-human beings, as in the case of school food). Further, popular education seeks to build capacity for long-term, sustained community organizing for the benefit of students and the larger community and planet, rather than a one-time service-learning experience, for example. Popular education proposes that *students are powerful*. With a popular education approach, students could potentially lobby for higher quality, ethically and sustainably sourced food for themselves and for the future. They could create their own campaign to teach fellow students how to make healthier food choices at school. They could advocate for mindful eating practices. They could interrogate the commercialism that has crept into the school cafeteria and campus. In this sense, education is necessarily a generative and political process, rather than a passive, static, unilateral, or apolitical one in which teachers impart information to students who are empty receptacles.

To achieve these ends, popular education pedagogy is based on a circular model of roughly three stages. There are many examples of how this is implemented, and here we present one such model from Arnold and Burke (1983). The first stage is to "begin with reality" (Arnold and Burke 1983), a stage that asks us to begin with the material experiences of the students. Second, students are asked to reflect on, expand, and then theorize that reality. Third, students then begin to plan concrete, and ideally sustainable, action. This cycle is repeated: action/reflection/action. Popular education incorporates a variety of strategies in these three stages, with an emphasis on hands-on, experiential, active learning. We can imagine arts-based approaches as particularly powerful. Below, we will provide examples of how one might design a radically democratic school food curriculum designed with popular education principles as a foundation. It is of course important to note that the students themselves would have the major role in directing the types of inquiries and projects in the curriculum.

## EXAMPLES: SCHOOL, HOME, AND OFF CAMPUS

We shall draw our examples from how school lunch could be theorized in a school, an offsite restaurant for students on an open campus, and at home. Within a school, we will discuss food consumed there, which of course can be either prepared there or brought in as a sack lunch from home. Lunch prepared and consumed at a restaurant and at home has some differences that can inform how lunch can be part of that particular educational experience.

Three scenarios in these settings highlight similarities and differences in the lunch itself, the ties to the wider community and larger contextual issues, and how the lunch can be part of the curriculum of the particular educational arrangement. Each example contrasts the implicit or hidden curriculum of the lunch with what, drawing upon Dewey, Freire, and the broader tenets of popular education, can become an active, explicit, and connected part of the curriculum, thus making school lunch more than just a means of satisfying hunger by unreflective consumption of nutrients and calories.

Our first example is a typical public high school, perhaps located in a small town, where everyone in the town attends the school. A. G. Rud would visit such a school in the nearby county seat when he was dean in order to consult with the county's superintendents, and the meeting would include food procured at the cafeteria. For our purposes, this school is not an open campus, and thus the students went to a designated cafeteria, and ate lunch food provided there or they brought lunch from home and perhaps only bought a beverage. School lunches now can more readily resemble food found in a mall food court, such as taco and salad bars, rather than food ladled out uniformly to students in a line. This high school has a small salad bar, with iceberg lettuce, cucumber and tomato slices, carrots, celery, croutons, and a variety of salad dressings. Cheeseburgers, hamburgers, tater tots, fish sticks, chicken nuggets, and such round out the offerings.

This is what Arnold and Burke (1983) call the stage of beginning with reality or the actual experience of the students. The students do not have any real say in what they are served, it being determined in a central office, and perhaps even hired out to a food service corporation. Given that the "lunch period" is set and brief, how can we inject reflection upon such a routine meal presentation? How can students become more aware of what they are eating, where it came from, how it is prepared, and the myriad other factors that go into this institutional setting? And, too, if students come from homes that are unreflective about what they eat, how it is harvested, slaughtered, delivered, and prepared, how can we expect the students to want to know more? Obviously, it is easier to open one's mind in a smaller, progressive setting such as the lab school that John and Alice Dewey ran in the early 1900s, where students learned cooking through actually engaging in those tasks. School lunch in this larger high school setting is separated from the official curriculum, and connecting it to what is taught elsewhere is a challenge. Part of the problem is of course that the official curriculum does not likely include any discussion of school food. Parents, teachers, and students are not consulted on what will be served, nor is there any coordination between what is studied when and what students can eat. Perhaps this is asking too much given the many issues schools face daily. A nod toward a certain ethnic group on the menu during a holiday may be all that is or can be done, but there could be much more to learn here.

One aspect of eating in the school that could be exploited is the difference between lunches prepared at the school itself versus those brought from home. Food brought from home presumably is chosen and purchased by a parent or guardian. There are varying degrees in how parents or guardians respond to a child's taste. Some parents may be mindful of what they are putting in the sack, as they believe they will be judged by not only their child but other children and their parents, as well as teachers and other school personnel who monitor the lunch period. An extreme example of lunch surveillance has occurred a number of times; a young student's lunch is considered not nutritious and is either taken away or sent home uneaten (e. g., Seidl 2012).

Food purchased at school has a history too of course, but one that is not always for nutritional value or ecological sustainability. As with the

National School Lunch Act, a subsidy to the food industries by schools helped these industries, having little relevance to nutrition and sustainability. So first students should know the history in more detail than we sketched earlier. Just reading the National School Lunch Act would be an eye-opener for many students unaccustomed to the historical context out of which it arose.

Merely reading a 70-year old governmental document that enacted a change across the country may sound ordinary enough, but here it is explicit that the midday meal can be a curricular component. Once this is done, other connections could be made, to the sciences of how food comes to the table, to the economic factors in food production, and to various customs, rituals, and lore associated with food preparation, presentation, and consumption. Of course, these connections would have to be an intentional part of the curriculum for all students, and not just a few in, say, a special social studies course.

We have focused here on the secondary school, and perhaps its well-cited compartmentalization of the curriculum makes it not the ideal place for this kind of curricular and pedagogical experimentation and innovation. Ideally, students would have learned more about what they eat midday at a younger age, building on nascent lessons on nutrition and sustainability their parents or guardians may impart before they get to school. Of course, words imparted by a parent or guardian vary tremendously as does all of our relations with what we seek out to prepare and eat.

Homeschooling and thus home lunch preparation and consumption present particular circumstances and factors that counter a wider context for learning. A homeschooled child would seem to have more opportunity to focus on preparation of food and learning about cooking, but this of course varies by the individual circumstance. What is obvious is that lunch at home during a school day is likely not different than lunch on the weekend for a homeschooler. It may be carefully regulated and dispensed by a parent or be merely whatever is in the refrigerator on the second shelf, help yourself. Lunch for a homeschooler is both alive with possibilities for study and reflection while at the same time potentially being inert and resistant to these possibilities simply because it is consumed at home. Educational policy surrounding feeding children midday in institutions can only be explored, if at all, at a curricular distance. It simply does not affect the homeschooler, except if one were to study aspects of school finance.

A third variation is the open campus school. This can only occur at the high school where students are allowed to leave campus during the lunch hour. Like homeschooling, open campus lunches present fewer curricular opportunities. This is not because there is not much to say about restaurants or corporate fast food. It is because this experience is not widely shared. At A. G. Rud's daughter's open campus high school in Indiana, students who went off campus could walk to several local restaurants and fast food chains, while some, with vehicles, could venture even further. One could learn about how restaurants compete and how they deliver their food to make profit, but none of that is unique to midday eating at school, much how a homeschooler consuming a parentally prepared sandwich at noon is not different from what may happen on the weekend for any child, homeschooled or not.

## CONCLUSION

We can see how theories based upon Dewey and Freire, as well as popular education as related to Freire, form a theoretical frame and context for considering school lunch as part of the curriculum. What is the likelihood that such a framing will result in the development of such a curriculum? We are mostly skeptical, but still hopeful. Dewey the progressive and Freire the radical have not fared well in terms of making significant change in mainstream education in America. Dewey's idea of a progressive, child-centered education focused on preparing youth for creative democratic engagement has been countered by routine teacher-centered instruction and the accountability/assessment emphasis in schools that focus on measurable results. Freire's ideas for popular education—ideas geared toward the education of Brazil's poor—have fared even worse. If we grant that this is the case for our chosen theorists, what value do our ideas have about connecting midday eating to curricular activities already in place? We can only continue to insist that midday eating on school days, whether at home, at school, or at a restaurant, provide opportunities to reflect upon food production, preparation, and consumption. These aspects of midday eating on school days deserve a place at the curricular table, joined to other facets of instruction and character formation typical in educational settings. If not, school lunch remains an untapped part of the school day for curricular integration and learning.

186    A. G. RUD AND S. GLEASON

# References

Arnold, R., & Burke, B. (1983). *A popular education handbook: An educational experience taken from Central America and adapted to the Canadian context.* Ottawa: CUSO Development Education.

Arteaga, I., & Heflin, C. (2014). Participation in the National School Lunch Program and food security: An analysis of transitions into kindergarten. *Children and Youth Services Review, 47,* 224–230.

Clark, M. A., & Fox, M. K. (2009). Nutritional quality of the diets of US public school children and the role of the school meal programs. *Journal of the American Dietetic Association, 109*(2), S44–S56.

De Lissovoy, N. (2010). Decolonial pedagogy and the ethics of the global. *Discourse: Studies in the Cultural Politics of Education, 31*(3), 279–293.

DeLeon, A. (2011). What's that nonhuman doing on your lunch tray: Disciplinary spaces, school cafeterias, and possibilities for resistance. In S. Robert & M. Weaver-Hightower (Eds.), *School food politics: The complex ecology of hunger and feeding in schools around the world* (pp. 183–200). New York: Peter Lang.

Freire, P. (2002). *Pedagogy of the oppressed.* New York: Continuum.

Huang, J., & Barnidge, E. (2016). Low-income children's participation in the National School Lunch Program and household food insufficiency. *Social Science & Medicine, 150*(C), 8–14.

JDKI Tenets. (2017). Retrieved from https://learn.uvm.edu/program/john-dewey-kitchen-institute/tenets/

John Dewey Kitchen Institute. (2017). Retrieved from https://learn.uvm.edu/program/john-dewey-kitchen-institute/

Kunzman, R. (2009). *Write these laws on your children: Inside the world of conservative Christian homeschooling.* Boston: Beacon Press.

Laird, S. (2008). Food for co-educational thought. In B. Stengel (Ed.), *Philosophy of education 2007* (pp. 1–13). Urbana: Philosophy of Education Society.

Levenstein, H. A. (1988). *Revolution at the table: The transformation of the American diet.* New York/Oxford: Oxford University Press.

Levenstein, H. A. (1993). *Paradox of plenty: A social history of eating in modern America.* New York/Oxford: Oxford University Press.

Miller, G. F., Gupta, S., Kropp, J. D., Grogan, K. A., & Mathews, A. (2016). The effects of pre-ordering and behavioral nudges on National School Lunch Program participants' food item selection. *Journal of Economic Psychology, 55,* 4–16.

Poppendieck, J. (2013). The ABCs of school lunch. In P. Pringle (Ed.), *A place at the table: The crisis of 49 million hungry Americans and how to solve it* (pp. 123–134). New York: Public Affairs.

Rowe, B., & Rocha, S. (2015). School lunch is not a meal: Posthuman eating as folk phenomenology. *Educational Studies, 51*(6), 482–496.

Rud, A. G. (2013). Midday eating while learning: The school cafeteria, home-schooling, and the open campus high school. *Journal of Thought, 48*(2), 78–88.

Seidl, J. M. (2012, February 12). *N. C. food "inspector" sends girl's lunch home after determining it's not healthy enough.* Retrieved from http://www.theblaze.com/news/2012/02/14/n-c-food-inspector-sends-girls-lunch-home-after-determining-its-not-healthy-enough/

Terry-McElrath, Y. M., O'Malley, P. M., & Johnston, L. D. (2015). Foods and beverages offered in US public secondary schools through the National School Lunch Program from 2011–2013: Early evidence of improved nutrition and reduced disparities. *Preventive Medicine, 78*, 52–58.

Zellner, D. A., & Cobuzzi, J. L. (2016). Just dessert: Serving fruit as a separate "dessert" course increases vegetable consumption in a school lunch. *Food Quality and Preference, 48*, 195–198.

Ziegelman, J. (2010). *97 Orchard: An edible history of five immigrant families in one New York tenement.* New York: Smithsonian Books/Harper Collins.

CHAPTER 11

# We Are How We Eat: An Argument for the Social Value of Slow School Lunch

*Jennifer C. Ng*

Several years ago, I led a study of how Bishop Seabury Academy, a private school in Lawrence, Kansas, does lunch (Ng et al. 2013). Established in 1997 with just 32 students, six teachers, and one Headmaster, Seabury now enrolls almost 180 students in grades 6–12 and has a staff of 28 teachers and administrators. From the school's very beginning, it has structured lunch to include all students and staff sitting together on Mondays, Tuesdays, and Thursdays in assigned, mixed-age arrangements that change every two weeks throughout the year. On Wednesdays, students sit with their *altera familias* or faculty advisors and mixed-grade advisory groups that remain constant from the time they enter Seabury to the time they graduate. On Fridays, all students get to choose where—and with whom—they want to sit, and seniors have the option of leaving the campus entirely.

Recognizing that school lunch involves not only the consumption of food but also the interactions of people gathered together in the lunch room at lunchtime, our primary interest in this earlier study of Seabury was to explore the potential of human relations education during lunch. A "human relations" approach, as Sleeter and Grant (2009) explain, refers to efforts that encourage the interaction of individuals who might

J. C. Ng (✉)
University of Kansas, Lawrence, KS, USA

© The Author(s) 2018                                                                 189
S. Rice, A. G. Rud (eds.), *Educational Dimensions of School Lunch*,
https://doi.org/10.1007/978-3-319-72517-8_11

otherwise lead quite separate social existences. These separations can be caused by—and reinforced through—biases, stereotypes, and prejudices. Moreover, opportunities for meaningful interaction with others across existing group boundaries can help people overcome barriers of difference and foster empathy, respect, and a shared sense of humanity instead.

Though there have been some changes over the years, Bishop Seabury's unique and longstanding practice of lunch made it an ideal setting for our exploration. The school now serves catered food in a buffet rather than family-style arrangement, and it uses a computer program developed by a former student to generate the biweekly seating assignments instead of having a staff member create them manually. The addition of sixth graders in 2011 to the previously existing 7–12 grade school boosted enrollment by 10 percent and prompted practical questions about whether the school's lunches could continue being accommodated in its existing space. Yet, broad support from staff and students, as well as the reconfiguration of tables in an expanded space called "The Commons," has ensured the continuation of this tradition into the foreseeable future.

Through observations during lunch and in-depth interviews with select school staff members and focus groups with students across all grades, our study ultimately illustrated that lunch *can* be conceived of as more than just a time to eat. Seabury lunches fostered feelings of school-wide community. Rather than conclude our study with the usual recommendations of how other schools could replicate Seabury's approach, however, we wondered whether readers would even share our appreciation for it. Returning to this question in the present chapter, I develop a critical examination of school lunch in its more conventional and taken-for-granted form. What is the character of our social engagement over food? What can be gained by drawing conceptually from the "slow" movement and the serious reconsideration of school lunch's potential, as realized through the example of Bishop Seabury?

## EATING AWAY AT LUNCHTIME

In 1825, the legendary French food writer, Anthelme Brillat-Savarin, noted that "the destiny of nations depends upon the manner in which they feed themselves" (Honore 2004, p. 57). And in 2001, journalist Eric Schlosser (2001) notoriously deemed the United States a "fast food nation." This characterization provokes reflection on not only the origin, taste, and nutritional value of the foods we consume. It expressly emphasizes that *how* we consume food is revealing. As Alice Waters (2006) elaborates,

When we pledge our dietary allegiance to a fast-food nation, there are also grave consequences to the health of our civil society and our national character. When we eat fast-food meals alone in our cars, we swallow the values and assumptions of the corporations that manufacture them. According to these values, eating is no more important than fueling up, and should be done quickly and anonymously.

Studies of "opportunity time to eat"—the time difference between a student's receipt of his or her lunch and the end of the lunch period (University of Washington School of Public Health 2015, p. 11)—suggest that school lunch is no exception to a fast food mentality. Indeed, the time allocated to eating itself is being eaten away. Many schools fall short of providing the minimum 20 minutes recommended by the National Alliance for Nutrition and Activity and the American Academy of Pediatrics. While a national survey conducted by the School Nutrition Association found that elementary school students have 25 minutes for lunch on average, accounting for the time it takes to go to the restroom, wash hands, walk to the cafeteria, and stand in line for meals, it means students are often left with only 10–15 minutes to eat (Hellmich 2011).

The challenge of allocating time for lunch further illustrates other related dilemmas. Forty percent of the nation's public schools start serving lunch by 10:45 a.m., and some schools begin at 9:25 a.m. because they are especially large or ill equipped to prepare food on such a scale (University of Washington School of Public Health 2015, p. 12). When recess follows lunch, students also rush to get outside—discarding less processed whole foods for options that require less chewing (Price and Just 2015). This daily practice of "rapid eating" results in food waste and lost opportunities for nutritional enrichment, which are individual as well as environmental and public health concerns. Children condition themselves to eat faster overall and miss normal bodily cues signaling their fullness (Buergel et al. 2002)—a bodily transformation that parallels a fast society's inclination toward becoming velocitized, or acclimated and endlessly desirous of more speed (Honore 2004).

The ensuing mentality that prioritizes fast food—or food fast—means that time for lunch continues to be up for grabs. In an era where the leisurely roots of a liberal education (Smile 2013) have been uprooted by the "learnification" of education (Biesta 2009), an increasingly important distinction is also what constitutes instructional time from all that is seemingly *non*-instructional time in schools. A recent story of parent protests in Wichita, Kansas, exemplifies the issue: The district's prescribed schedule includes 4.5 hours of reading and math instruction with several "uninterrupted blocks" for core curriculum and additional intensive instruction for students performing below grade level. Additional weekly requirements for social studies, science, health, music, physical education, library, and art—as well as nearly four hours of teacher planning time—leave little time for recess. Yet, educators recognize students need "brain breaks."

To preserve instructional time and allow students these necessary breaks, Wichita school leaders sought to maximize the efficiency of student eating by silencing talking at lunch. The principal of Price-Harris Elementary School described the "voice level zero" approach to lunch as reasonable and necessary. He explained, "We ask [students] to stay at zero [talking] because otherwise they're not really paying attention. It takes longer to get through the line, they have less time to eat, and they have less time to play" (Tobias 2016).

Just as this example from Wichita makes clear, the "time troubles" of school lunch are not remedied merely by assigning more minutes to it (Poppendieck 2010). Slowing the fast pace of school lunch is not simply about chewing less hastily, either. What must be central in our consideration is whether we conceive of lunch as a time for anything at all worthwhile. Are there educational lessons extending from lunch that are not only nutritional but also social? What are the "slow food values" exemplified in the traditional family meal "which teaches us, among other things, that the pleasures of the table are a social as well as a private good[?]" As Waters (2006) points out, it is "at the table we learn moderation, conversation, tolerance, generosity and conviviality…".

## BITING BACK FOR SOMETHING BETTER

It is a sad reality that not every child eats his or her lunch in a safe, welcoming, and inclusive setting. Researchers have amply detailed the lunch room at lunchtime as an important site of peer interaction, identity formation, and status differentiation (Adler and Adler 1995; Bishop et al. 2004; Kinney 1993). They have also emphasized that the resulting friendship circles or cliques in a cafeteria are influenced by such things as race (Tatum 2003), class (Eckert 1989), gender and age (Eder 1995), and other manifestations of difference (Milner 2006). Nevertheless, the warm publicity generated by a photo that recently went viral of Travis Randolph, a Florida State University football player, sitting with Bo Paske, a 11-year-old middle schooler with autism who usually eats lunch alone, reveals the resigned acceptance that otherwise seems to exist toward the social dynamics of lunch (Chan 2016). The Teaching Tolerance campaign to "Mix It Up at Lunch" is one popular initiative meant to improve the social dynamics of lunch. Involving more than 2500 students at schools in the United States and abroad (Severson 2012), a featured aspect of Mix It Up programming is for students to sit with classmates different from their usual lunchtime company for one day (Willoughby 2011). Little research has been done about these efforts or their impact, though. In one of the few studies available, Kindzierski et al. (2013) found that third graders who participated at two different elementary schools felt uncomfortable and reported little to no connection with their randomly assigned classmates after the day's experience of mixed lunch. The majority of students thought the activity was "okay" or said they "like it," but they also described "barely talking" or "talking about nothing really." Overwhelmingly, they preferred that things "stay the way they are" at their schools.

A free, lunch-planning app called "Sit with Us" invented by an 11th grader in 2016 similarly reinforces the point that the cruel, daily circumstances of lunch so many students face must be changed. Yet, it importantly highlights how such change must be deliberate. Born out of her personal experiences of being bullied and sitting alone for the entirety of her seventh-grade year at an all-girls school (Love 2016), the app's inventor, Natalie Hampton, explained on National Public Radio's *All Things Considered*:

> When you walk into the lunchroom and you see all the tables and everyone sitting there. You know that going up to them would only end in rejection, you feel extremely alone and extremely isolated, and your stomach drops. And you are searching for a place to eat, but you know that if you sit by yourself, there'll be so much embarrassment that comes with it because people will know and they'll see you as the girl who has nowhere to sit.

Natalie Hampton attends a new school where she is personally "thriving" now, but the lunchroom dynamics of social exclusion exist there as well. Wanting to "stand up and do something about all the kids who feel [left out] every day," she designed an app where students can sign up to become ambassadors in their schools and post seats in the cafeteria available to anyone who needs a place to sit. The high-tech nature of the app is essential, she insisted, because "I tried many times to reach out to someone, but I was rejected many times. ...This way it's very private. It's through the phone. No one else has to know. And you know that you're not going to be rejected once you get to the table" (National Public Radio 2016).

Whereas secrecy is a key component of Hampton's app, Seabury's lunchtime routines are a publicly visible display of the school's efforts to normalize inclusion. One staff member described Seabury's use of mixed-age assigned seating at lunch as a "different, very creative, and very in tune with an adolescents' psyche" way to counter their seemingly inevitable tendencies toward cliquish behavior. Another teacher noted, too, the reputation of teachers' lounges during lunchtime as places where adults could isolate themselves from students to complain or be catty with their colleagues. "I don't talk about my students. If I have an issue with a student, I'll just go and speak to the student candidly, you know? I don't gossip about my students."

Consistent with the popular media portrayals and likely the life experiences of many people, one teacher recalled her own high school lunch period as being fraught with anxiety. She recalled, "It was a stressful time of my day. I was worried, who would sit with me? Would my friends be there? Or, would I be, you know, carrying my tray hoping someone was going to let me sit at their table?" In contrast, the belief underlying Seabury's explicit premise for inclusion was voiced by its Headmaster who said, "It's the separation that breeds disrespect, lack of empathy." The resulting experience of lunch at Seabury, then, was captured by a student who explained,

> You don't have to worry about, 'Oh my gosh, my friend is sitting over here. I'm going to sit over there.' And if someone wants to sit with you, at my old school my friends would be like, 'I'll sit with you, but there are no seats left.' So, they would feel sad, they would feel bad. They would feel discluded, and this way no one feels discluded [sic].

The degree of daily variety balanced by "a good sameness" of overall expectations was meant to safeguard students against feelings of fear, concern, or apprehension about lunch, a staff person emphasized. And if on Fridays students formed groups that excluded certain individuals, the Headmaster was clear: "We go back to doing [lunch by assignment every day] because there is a responsibility on all levels." When this happened once among students in the sixth grade, they were temporarily not allowed to choose their seats again and sat together as a single group of sixth graders instead. According to the Headmaster, readings on community and conversations about "What happened? Why did it happen? Who's excluded? Why did you do this? How did it make them feel? Have you ever been excluded? What's going on?" became part of the text of the class.

Seabury's varied lunch formats afforded all members of the school opportunities for comparison through their contrasting experiences. This was already the case for staff and students who could recall the dynamics of schools they had previously worked in or attended. But reflection upon the range of existing and other possible practices seemed to heighten shared appreciation for Seabury's approach. Critical to Seabury's effectiveness were the normalization of social interaction through formal policies and procedures; the close integration of lunch and other school-wide efforts to build community; and a strategic reconceptualization of individual choice exercised through the process of learning at lunch.

## TRAINING AT THE TROUGH

When lunch functions primarily as a pause for refueling the body during a day otherwise designed to school the mind, then its potential as an educationally relevant time is squandered (Weaver-Hightower 2011). What we observed in the efforts of school staff at Bishop Seabury, however, was the deliberate reconciliation of body and mind at lunch to promote positive social interaction. As the Headmaster explained, "One of the things we tell [students is that their job at the table], when you eat, when you're with people...it is a place for discussion. You are doing two things with your mouth at once. It is a place to share ideas, to build community."

Without the shared speech that fosters community among diners, Kass argues, "the belly rules the mouth, and the table becomes no different than a trough" (as cited by Smilie 2013, p. 62). So asking students to make something more of lunch than might be typically imagined means an ongoing training of students' expectations, behaviors, and values at the metaphorical trough must be deliberately initiated. Training in this sense is not about the generic development of skills premised on universal prescriptions of "best practice" and "what works." Rather, it is the sort of training exercised by a gardener in the slow art of bonsai—a purposeful orientation of growth that relates a subject and its environment in accordance with a guiding vision. It expresses a definite philosophical position, it draws on tradition and character, and it is about moral choices (Holt 2002).

Through direct instruction, modeling, and gentle reminders as needed, Seabury students did more than consume food together. They collectively paused for daily prayer, stood to acknowledge the arrival of adult staff or guests at the table, asked for the salt and pepper to be passed rather than reaching across others, and showed self-awareness about potentially inappropriate behavior, such as playing with their food. Students attributed the development of these manners as well as a mindfulness about cleaning up after themselves and wanting to behave in an acceptable way to Seabury lunches. And, when asked hypothetically for their reactions to an announcement that Seabury students would now be able to choose who they wanted to sit with every day just as students normally do in other schools, one student replied, "I think if that were to happen, the meek and timid people who don't have anyone to sit with at lunch time would form an impromptu revolution on the school and on the Headmaster's office to demand [our] normal lunches back."

## Hungering for a Complete Conversation

Students recalled being "surprised," "confused," or "scared" when they first learned about Seabury's mixed-age assigned seating practice at lunch. Some thought it would be "weird" while others thought it was an "interesting" idea and something "new" to try. One student remembered, "I thought [the school was] making a big deal out of something that wasn't." Yet, like all the students we spoke to, this student ultimately came to appreciate lunch at Seabury and described it as more like eating dinner than lunch—something with bigger expectations, sitting down, and social time. Another student memorably called the social time afforded by lunch a chance to have a "complete conversation" threading through what might have started during the day's school-wide morning meeting, advisory group, class, or some other point.

The goals associated with lunch at Seabury so thoroughly permeated other aspects of the day that the Headmaster paused when asked what difference he thought lunches might have made on individual students. "I tend to think of it as a composite between altera familia in the morning, morning meeting, and lunch," he realized. "I tend to see it grouped together, so maybe I'm talking about more than just lunch." Several students and staff members actually insisted that lunches at Seabury were synonymous with the school itself. Descriptors of lunch as "safe," "welcoming," and "family"-like thus referred to the broader environment of the school as well.

One staff person distinguished lunch as unique from other times of the school day, however, because lunchtime afforded people opportunities to get acquainted as individuals rather than such singular categories as "teacher," "senior," "international student," or "newbie." "At that lunch table," she said, "you are just someone having lunch with someone else." Another teacher agreed, "We are outside the classroom, and we are interacting as people. People that are just at different stages of our lives."

Lunches themselves could function only as opportunities for engagement, one staff person noted. And students recognized that the quality of resulting exchanges depended on the participation of all individuals. "Good" tables were characterized as having adult leaders who set a tone for the group's involvement by asking open-ended and stimulating questions. "Bad" tables, which were fortunately a "rare occasion" according to upperclassmen, were those where conversation seemed awkward, contrived, or almost non-existent. In these instances, many students indicated their willingness to step up and test their conversational abilities. Students described these abilities as having developed over time and with both guidance and continued practice,

I think 6th graders are really shy for about a week and don't really want to talk to anybody, but I think the older kids try to include you. I think it just took us awhile. (Sixth grade focus group)

Teachers kind of lead...but the students help to set an example for the younger kids. Last year, I did not know what to do at lunch, but the students would start talking and look at you, and you though, I better start talking or I will look like an idiot. So, it is like helping out your friends to know how to do this. (Grades 7–8 focus group)

Like when you're a 6th grader, if you don't have to talk to a senior, you're probably not going to but then when it's like thrust upon you, not in a bad way, but like you're going to sit with a senior and a bunch of other grades, they are going to ask you questions and they are going to talk to you. I think it helps, like 6th graders and 7th graders become more comfortable around older kids in general. (Ninth and Tenth grade focus group)

And,

I think [mixed lunches] benefit international students more than other students because they're afraid to speak English and are more shy. So, it's more success for international students. (International student focus group)

Upperclassmen had the longest range perspective, recounting,

> Student 1: After you get older, you realize how helpful [lunch] was.
> Student 2: I don't think we really reflect every day on what lunch is doing.
> Student 3: Yeah, this is the first time we've really thought about it...
> Student 4: Before now, I just thought about it as eating lunch with a bunch of people. But now looking back on it, I realize that there was a reason. (11th–12th grade focus group)

The awareness students described as emerging through the years highlighted a Seabury teacher's point that "every lunch [counts] toward something."

## MAKING CHOICES WORTH WANTING

Across staff- and student-respondents alike, there was clarity expressed about the purposes of Seabury's approach to lunch and support for its implementation. Teachers referred to their commitment in terms of having "drunk the Kool-Aid" or being "all in," and the Headmaster concluded, "I am absolutely certain that this is the best way I can think of right now to have lunches." The only thing that could affect this conviction, he indicated, was,

> If you talk to students and you hear, 'Well, I look forward to Fridays [and just choosing who I sit with]. And, [teachers] say we [engage everyone], but we don't really do it. I don't understand why we do it, and there are always side conversations. The teachers at my table generally don't take any interest.' If I heard that, I wouldn't change lunches, I would start talking to the kids...

To the school's credit, students we spoke to at Bishop Seabury also expressed wanting things to stay the same at their school. Their comments were generally quite positive and included feelings of gratitude for "teachers [who] include you so much" and have made lunch "how it should be." One student in the grades 7–8 focus group explained, "We are forced into the best way to meet people. We can meet teachers without other kids thinking you are weird for walking to talk to them or meet them." An international student added, "For me, I not feel comfortable to make opportunity by myself to make friends or to get familiar with other people, so the assignment table is like a way to force me to make friends with others. It is a good opportunity for me."

Through their experiences of lunch at Seabury, students reconceived of "choice" as something they did not know they wanted, or as something they needed to learn they liked and then would have freely chosen. The productive tension within this new understanding of freedom and choice strengthened the effectiveness of Seabury's approach. As one student put it, "[If I had the chance], I would tell [my parents and teachers] how cool it is to sit with who I want...kind of who I want even if I didn't choose. You end up kind of wanting to sit with the people you end up sitting with." Conceiving of Seabury's lunches in terms of Howe's (1992) notion of cultivating "strong" freedom and opportunities "worth wanting," students were provided both structured experiences—from which inclusion was an explicit premise—to deliberate meaningfully about lunch practices and then also the chance to exercise their resulting choices in social conditions sheltered from the burden of scrutiny imposed by others.

A few students suggested Seabury's approach to lunch was something they could imagine sustaining on their own if ever the formal protocols were changed, and every day became a free-choice Friday. One student in the grades 7–8 focus group said tentatively, "I might choose to sit with someone I did not know, but maybe not with someone three years older than me." Another asserted more confidently, "I would sit with someone I did not know and had not sat with during assigned seating during the year. Sure, why not?" The only request he had for improving the existing system was to make the completely randomized generation of seat assignments strategically more deliberate.

> Last year, you could ask to sit with someone you had not sat with yet by the end of the year, and it would happen because [a person] organized and sorted the names. But this year, the assignments are sorted by a [computer] program, so you can't ask to sit with a teacher you haven't sat with. Can you please make this happen?

## CONCLUSION

We wanted to study Seabury because of its particular approach to lunch, and through our exploration we found it to be exceptional both in terms of it being quite excellent and in terms of it being quite rare. Students showed a maturity of sorts that one teacher related figuratively to a sweater that is created stich by stitch through the slow work of knitting and meant for a loved one to wear.

> We push it, we push it, we push it. We control it, control it, control it. But once you get to be a certain age, everything that we've been trying to tell you and teach you, you go, 'Okay. That's a sweater I'll put on for myself. You've shown me that sweater. You've made me wear that sweater. And now I realize that's a good sweater. Now I'm going to wear it.'

If through the practice of slow school lunch students can learn the value of such a metaphorical sweater, then perhaps there is hope that we can all come to appreciate Mahatma Gandhi's larger point that "there is more to life than increasing its speed" (as cited in Honore 2004).

## REFERENCES

Adler, P. A., & Adler, P. (1995). Dynamics of inclusion and exclusion in preadolescent cliques. *Social Psychology Quarterly, 58*(3), 145–162.

Biesta, G. (2009). Good education in an age of measurement: On the need to reconnect with the question of purpose in education. *Educational Assessment, Evaluation, and Accountability, 21*, 33–46.

Bishop, J. H., Bishop, M., Bishop, M., Gelbwasser, L., Green, S., Peterson, E., Rubinsztaj, A., & Zuckerman, A. (2004). Why we harass nerds and freaks: A formal theory of student culture norms. *Journal of School Health, 7*(7), 235–251.

Buergel, N. S., Bergman, E. A., Knutson, A. C., & Lindaas, M. A. (2002). Students consuming sack lunches devote more time to eating than those consuming school lunches. *Journal of the American Dietetic Association, 102*(9), 1283–1286.

Chan, M. (2016). Boy with autism who ate lunch with football player no longer sits alone. *Time*. Retrieved from http://time.com/4478169/boy-autism-football-player-fsu-travis-rudolph-lunch-alone/

Eckert, P. (1989). *Jocks and burnouts: Social categories and identity in the high school*. New York: Teachers College Press.

Eder, D. (1995). *School talk: Gender and adolescent culture*. New Brunswick: Rutgers University Press.

Hellmich, N. (2011). Cutting short lunch time in school may lead to obesity. *USA Today*. Retrieved from http://usatoday30.usatoday.com/news/health/wellness/story/2011/08/Students-feel-rushed-at-school-lunch/

Holt, M. (2002). It's time to start the slow school movement. *Phi Delta Kappan, 84*(4), 264–271.

Honore, C. (2004). *In praise of slowness: Challenging the cult of speed.* New York: Harper Collins Publishers.

Howe, K. R. (1992). Equal educational opportunity, and the challenge of multiculturalism. *American Educational Research Journal, 29*(3), 455–470.

Kindzierski, C. M., Leavitt-Noble, K., Dutt-Doner, K., Marable, M. A., & Wallace, N. (2013). Teaching tolerance with Mix It Up! Student reactions to an unusual lunch period. *Childhood Education, 89*(1), 15–18.

Kinney, D. A. (1993). From nerds to normal: The recovery of identity among adolescents from middle school to high school. *Sociology of Education, 66*(1), 21–40.

Love, M. (2016, September 5). Sherman Oaks teen takes on bullying with kindness-based app. *LA Daily News.* Retrieved from http://www.dailynews.com/media/20160905/sherman-oaks-teen-takes-on-bullying-with-kindness-based-app

Milner, M. (2006). *Freaks, geeks, and cool kids.* New York: Routledge Press.

National Public Radio. (2016, September 9). Teen creates 'Sit with Us' app for bullied kids. *All Things Considered.* Retrieved from http://www.npr.org/2016/09/09/493319114/teen-creates-sit-with-us-app-for-bullied-kids

Ng, J., Sweeney, H. M., & Mitchiner, M. (2013, Summer). Let's sit together. Exploring the potential for human relations education at lunch. *Journal of Thought, 48*(2), 65–77.

Poppendieck, J. (2010). *Free for all: Fixing school food in America.* Berkeley: University California Press.

Price, J., & Just, D. R. (2015). Lunch, recess and nutrition: Responding to time incentives in the cafeteria. *Preventive Medicine, 71*, 27–30.

Schlosser, E. (2001). *Fast food nation: The dark side of the all-American meal.* New York: Penguin Press.

Severson, K. (2012, October 14). Christian group finds gay agenda in anti-bullying day. *The New York Times.* Retrieved from http://www.nytimes.com

Sleeter, C. E., & Grant, C. A. (2009). *Making choices for multicultural education: Five approaches to race, class, and gender.* Hoboken: John Wiley & Sons.

Smilie, K. D. (2013, Summer). Time to eat: School lunch and the loss of leisure in education. *Journal of Thought, 48*(2), 49–64.

Tatum, B. D. (2003). *Why are all the black kids sitting together in the cafeteria?* New York: Basic Books.

Tobias, S. P. (2016, March 4). Wichita parents fight for kids' right to recess. *The Wichita Eagle.* Retrieved from http://www.kansas.com/news/local/education/articles63924492.html

University of Washington School of Publich Health. (2015, March). *Lunch time at school: How much is enough? An assessment of school lunch seat-time in Seattle public schools.* Seattle: Nutritional Sciences Program.

Waters, A. (2006). Slow food nation. *The Nation*. Retrieved from https://www.thenation.com/article/slow-food-nation/

Weaver-Hightower, M. B. (2011). Why education researchers should take school food seriously. *Educational Researcher, 40*(1), 15–21.

Willoughby, B. (2011, October 20). *Mix It Up at Lunch: So what's next?* Retrieved from http://www.tolerance.org/blog/mix-it-lunch-so-what-s-next

# INDEX[1]

[1] Note: Page numbers followed by 'n' denotes note.

© The Author(s) 2018
S. Rice, A. G. Rud (eds.), *Educational Dimensions of School Lunch*,
https://doi.org/10.1007/978-3-319-72517-8

Slow Food movement, the, 15
slow food values, 192
Smilie, Kipton, 7, 195
Smith, Neil, 13, 21
Social and Health Research Center,
the, 64
Social justice, ix, 2, 12, 94–96, 107, 162
Social networking
and lunchrooms, 137, 138, 145
technological, 111
Social sciences, 13, 127, 157
Social security, 102
Social spaces, 145
lunchrooms as, 7, 40, 145
Social welfare, 64, 103, 109
school lunch as, 37
Socrates, 53, 54
Somalia, 102
Southern Poverty Law Center
(SPLC), 152
Special education (SPED), 7, 8, 136,
143, 148, 149, 159
and school lunch policy, 135–153
Special Milk Program, 64
Stapleton, Sarah Riggs, x, 8
Steiner, Rudolf, ix, 13, 28
Sterilization, 142
Subway, 46, 65
Surveillance
lunch surveillance, 5, 64–70, 183
lunchtime policy as, 60, 61
Sustainability
education, 22
nutrition and, 174–176, 183, 184
Swan, Elaine, 60, 61
Sweeney, Holly Morsbach, 197

T
Tatum, Beverly Daniel, 140, 141, 192
Taubman, Peter M., 80, 84, 85

Technologies of power, 36–43
Thorne, Barrie, 136, 137, 141,
145, 146
*Three Thousand Years of Educational
Wisdom*, 23
*Title IX of the Education Amendments
of 1972*, 18
Topeka Psychoanalytic
Society, 77–80, 82
Transitional objects, 76
Trevino, Robert, 64

U
Ulich, Robert, 23
United Kingdom (UK), the, ix, 59,
60, 64, 66, 67
*The United States of Arugula*, 26
U.S. Bureau of Labor Statistics, 103
U.S. Department of Agriculture
(USDA), 19, 64, 92, 102, 103,
158, 166
United States National Research
Council, 75
*Universal Declaration of Human
Rights* (UDHR), 92, 101, 102
University of California State,
Davis, 103
University of California-Berkeley, 19
University of Chicago
Department of Philosophy and
Pedagogy, 13
Laboratory School, 13, 15
University of Paris, 19
University of Vermont, the, 177

V
*Vindication of the Rights of Woman,
A*, 17
Voice level zero, 192